SEXUAL HEALTH FOR MEN

The 'at your fingertips' guide

Dr Philip Kell MB, BS, FRCOG, FRCP(I), MFFP, FACSHP, MBA, MSc
*Consultant Physician, Archway Sexual Health Clinic, London;
Honorary Senior Lecturer, Academic Department of STDs, UCL;
Consultant Physician at St John's and St Elizabeth's Hospital,
London*

Vanessa Griffiths
*Nurse Consultant – Sexual Health, Nottingham; Honorary Lecturer,
Nottingham and Warwick*

CLASS PUBLISHING • LONDON

The authors assert their right as set out in Sections 77 and 78 of the Copyright Designs and Patents Act 1988 to be identified as the authors of this work wherever it is published commercially and whenever any adaptation of this work is published or produced including any sound recordings or films made of or based upon this work.

Printing history
First published 2003

The authors and publishers welcome feedback from the users of this book. Please contact the publishers.

Class Publishing, Barb House, Barb Mews, London W6 7PA, UK
Telephone: 020 7371 2119
Fax: 020 7371 2878 [International +4420]
email: post@class.co.uk
Visit our website – www.class.co.uk

616.69
KEL

A CIP catalogue for this book is available from the British Library

ISBN 1 85959 011 X

Edited by Michèle Clarke

Cartoons by Jane Taylor

Line illustrations by David Woodroffe

Indexed by Valerie Elliston

Typeset by Martin Bristow

Printed and bound in Finland by WS Bookwell, Juva

Contents

Acknowledgements

We should like to thank the following for their time and thoughtful suggestions on the content of the early manuscript: Ann Tailor of the Sexual Dysfunction Association (formerly the Impotence Association); Barbara Doyle of Owen Mumford and Bob Smith and his wife Pat, who, as well as reviewing the book for us, also agreed to be on our cover. Bob Smith has suffered with sexual dysfunction for 15 years owing to a spinal and nerve injury.

We would also like to thank the various authors of other Class Health publications who kindly gave permission for some of their questions and answers to be used: Dr Graham Jackson, author of *Heart Health – the 'at your fingertips' guide*; Dr Marie Oxtoby and Professor Adrian Williams, authors of *Parkinson's – the 'at your fingertips' guide*; Professor Peter Sönksen, Dr Charles Fox and Sue Judd, authors of *Diabetes – the 'at your fingertips' guide*; Dr Andy Stein and Janet Wild, authors of *Kidney Failure Explained*; Dr Julian Tudor Hart, Dr Tom Fahey and Professor Wendy Savage, authors of *High Blood Pressure – the 'at your fingertips' guide*; Professor Ian Robinson, Dr Stuart Neilson and Dr Frank Clifford Rose, authors of *Multiple Sclerosis – the 'at your fingertips' guide*.

Thanks also to the publishing team: Dick Warner who chivvied me so politely to finish the text, to Michèle Clarke who patiently rearranged and edited the text, to Jane Taylor for her naughty rabbits and to Emily Hicks for her cool eye at the end.

Note to reader

There is a glossary at the end of this book to help you with any words that may be unfamiliar to you. If you are looking for particular topics, you can use either the detailed list of Contents on pages v–vii or the Index, which starts on page 165.

We do recommend that you research the problems of erectile dysfunction to gain a greater understanding of it. We advise throughout this book the need for good communication with your partner and your doctor but you may find that, although your doctor is sympathetic to your worries, he or she may not have any training in this area, and a referral to a specialist clinic would be better.

1
Sexual dysfunction explained

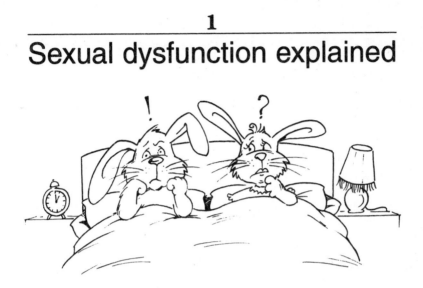

There are several aspects to sexual dysfunction – problems can range from difficulty in getting or maintaining an erection, to ejaculating too quickly or not being able to ejaculate at all. Problems with erection can be due to psychological or emotional instances, or simply an incompatibility between partners' needs and desires, or disease and illness and accidents causing damage to the body. We frequently get asked questions about possible impotence or other 'difficult' sexual problems. The ones below are some of the most common, and the following chapters enlarge on these questions.

My doctor keeps talking about sexual dysfunction. All I know is that I don't have sex any more with my girlfriend. So, what does sexual dysfunction actually mean?

The ability for two people to have equally satisfying sexual relations is one of the most important issues affecting quality of life. Sexual dysfunction is the medical term for the variety of problems occurring in men or women and which can affect sexual relations.

Sexual stimulation is an important process within the 'making love' process. The making love or sexual intercourse can be divided into an arousal phase, orgasm phase and a resolution phase. Problems can occur in any of these phases, although most commonly in the first and second.

In men, the more common problems concern 'erectile dysfunction' and 'rapid ejaculation'. These are explained below. In women it is loss of interest in sex and failure to achieve orgasm (anorgasmia). Painful intercourse (dyspareunia) happens in both men and women. It is more common in women but can occur in men, especially if they have a tight foreskin, if they have skin conditions that flare up with friction, or if they have candida (thrush) or herpes infections affecting their genitals. All these problems can cause what we call sexual dysfunction and we hope that the following chapters will help you find some answers to your questions.

I cannot get an erection at all at the moment. Will this mean that I shall always be impotent?

The definition of impotence, or erectile dysfunction (ED), as doctors and nurses now call it, is the 'persistent inability to obtain or maintain a penile erection that is sufficient to achieve the kind of sex you want with your partner.' There are several important parts of this definition:

- *obtaining an erection*: this is the ability to actually get the penis hard enough to be able to penetrate a partner;
- *maintaining an erection*: many men complain that they have no difficulty getting an erection, but the problem is maintaining it through intercourse, as their penises go limp (flaccid) prior to coming (ejaculation);
- *being persistently unable to have an erection*: at some stages of their lives, all men, or the vast majority at least, will have occasional problems with getting an erection

from excess stress, alcohol, tiredness or indeed many other factors, but you don't need to worry about this or even get treatment if it happens only occasionally.

However, if you feel your problem is affecting your quality of life, then some of the answers in this book might be able to help you. Your doctor will also be one of the best people to consult.

An erection does not have to be so hard that you can 'hang two wet towels on it', as the old saying goes, or last any specific length of time, but it should be hard enough and last long enough for both you and your partner to be satisfied with sex.

What are erections?

What actually is happening within my penis when I have an erection?

Erections are all about getting blood into the penis, so erections depend upon blood vessels and the nerves that control them. It is actually the opposite of what you might think. When the penis is limp, the blood vessels are active, and something called the sympathetic nervous system is mainly working. During sexual activity, the 'parasympathetic nervous system' takes over and the blood vessels relax and open up, allowing the blood to flow into the penis. The penis then fills with blood and this 'engorgement' blocks off the blood vessels that drain the blood away from the penis.

Within the penis, there are three tall columns of tissue: the largest two are on each side and are known as the corpora cavernosa. These are honeycomb-like structures, which fill with blood when there is sexual stimulation. The third one is the middle part, which is called the corpus spongiosum, and this contains the urethra, or the tube that passes through the penis from the bladder, through which men both urinate and ejaculate. The corpus spongiosum expands at the end of the penis to make the head of the penis or the glans. Figure 1.1 illustrates what is happening.

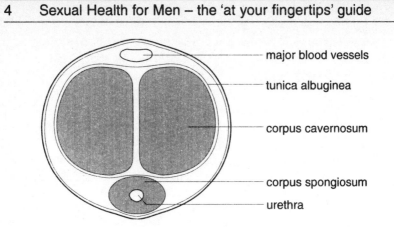

Figure 1.1 Cross-section of penis.

   Surrounding each of the two corpora cavernosa is a fibrous or tough layer of tissue called the 'tunica albuginea'. When the corpora fill with blood, this tunica stretches and blocks off the small blood vessels to prevent the blood leaking away. This so-called 'venous leakage' was thought previously to be an important cause of ED, and many men had surgery in order to repair it. However, it became clear that this surgery did not help men in the long term and hence it is not done as frequently as it once was.

Diagnosis of ED

If I do go to my doctor, would he be able to diagnose impotence? How would he know for sure? Surely only myself and my partner can know that?

There are no tests that can or should be done to confirm a diagnosis of impotence (erectile dysfunction). If you and/or your partner think that one of you has a problem, your doctor will understand your worry and will take a detailed history, then give you information about what you might be able to do. However, your doctor *will* do tests in order to find any serious illnesses that may be associated with your erection problems, such as tests to exclude diabetes (a blood or urine test) or cardiovascular problems (blood pressure and blood cholesterol levels). This might be the first time that you have visited your general practitioner in many years and, if this is the case, your doctor may use this as a good opportunity to do a general healthcare examination for you; for instance he might do tests to make sure that you haven't got prostate cancer, particularly if you are over 50.

At your consultation, the doctor will probably ask some specific questions about your sex life and, although this can be embarrassing, answering them correctly will help the doctor to come to correct decisions about possible treatment. Questions might include:

- *What actually happens when you try and have sex?*
- *How long has the problem being going on?*
- *Did you notice that the problem was sudden or had taken some time to develop?*
- *Is your partner aware that you are having problems with your erections?*
- *Do you ever have morning or spontaneous erections?*
- *Is this the first time you have consulted a doctor about the problem?*
- *Is your partner interested in joining in consultations or treatments?*
- *Have you any idea what might have started it all?*
- *What would you like the outcome to be from this visit?*

Examination

When I went to my doctor's he asked me lots of questions and then asked to see my penis. Why was this necessary? My problem starts when I'm having sex!

Your doctor will ask to make an examination of your genitals in order to see whether they are 'normal' in appearance – lots of men think that a 'small penis' is the root of all their problems. This is mostly a myth. Penis length has nothing to do with ED, but penis deformity might have. For example, very low levels of testosterone can be indicated by testicles that are difficult to find; a penis could be 'buried' by scrotal swelling, or the penis can be bent and painful in Peyronie's disease (see Chapter 12). Obesity also can cause apparent shortening of your penis, so your doctor will talk about possible diet changes to help you lose weight if you are overweight.

While you are there, your doctor will also examine your testicles, as a routine check for cancer.

Blood tests

I didn't think there was a specific test for ED. Why does my doctor want to do blood tests?

Blood tests can be very useful for indicating whether there are other disorders going on that might be causing your ED. Your doctor will test for diabetes, which is known to cause problems with blood supply or nerves and is a common cause of ED, or hormone deficiency (such as testosterone, low levels of which will affect your sex drive – libido). There is more about testosterone in Chapter 2. Your blood pressure will also be measured.

A check will also be made for any possible cardiovascular problems.

Symptoms

My girlfriend just doesn't seem interested in sex, which is making me very frustrated. What should I do?

If your partner is not as interested in having sex as often as you are, you need to talk to her about this issue and reach a compromise with which you can both live. Sex is all about communication. If you can communicate about sex, which is a key quality of life issue, your relationship will probably be all the better for it. Maybe your girlfriend is having problems herself, such as dyspareunia (see earlier question), or perhaps her feelings for you have changed. She may well be stressed or worried. You haven't mentioned whether you have children at home – they can have a big impact on a relationship! If you can talk about how you feel to her, maybe she will feel happier about talking things over with her doctor or even yourself.

It is well known that men and women have different timings throughout a month of sexual peaks and troughs. Getting them to coincide every time can be difficult but any stimulation with films, books, or even fantasy, could be the answer.

I can't maintain my erections long enough to satisfy my girlfriend. Does this mean that I am impotent?

The definition of impotence (erectile dysfunction) is a persistent inability to obtain or maintain an erection suitable for intercourse. All men will have intermittent erection problems from stress, tiredness or an excess of drugs or alcohol. Impotence from this sort of problem does not need 'medical' treatment and your erections will get better in time once the causes are recognized and dealt with.

Failure to get an erection means that your penis does not get hard enough to enable you to enter your partner. Not being able to keep an erection is a very common sexual problem, and is caused by the same factors that cause a failure to get one in the first place and is treated in the same manner.

You should see your doctor and discuss your situation with him to get a correct diagnosis and treatment in your case – and there are a variety of treatments on offer nowadays.

I am too tired at nights to bother with sex. This is upsetting my partner but my work is taking all my energy away.

In the modern world we all seem to suffer from stress and tiredness. One obvious way forward is to consider at what times you feel least tired – at the weekends perhaps. Rather than thinking of sexual intercourse as the major element, you could agree with your partner to engage in some other less energetic sexual activities – such as gentle stroking or foreplay – that you could participate in more frequently. Sometimes we can get stressed from being in the wrong job, although in today's economic climate this is not so easy. Plan your time between work and 'self-time' – sex cannot always be spontaneous, but 'foreplay' and talking with your partner can be planned.

Perhaps your partner's concern is not the lack of sex but the lack of intimacy. Sometimes, when men are not in the 'mood' for sex, all forms of intimacy stop, hence there may be no kissing, hugging, holding hands or even communication. You really need to talk together.

I can't get a hard penis at all, but am too embarrassed to tell anyone. I feel completely isolated and worthless. Am I the only man that this is happening to?

No! ED is a very common problem, particularly as men get older. There have been studies show that, in men over 50, up to 50% will have at least some problems with their erections and 1 in 10 men over the age of 40 will have problems due to age, regardless of any health problems. Several of your friends may have this problem, but might never have felt able to discuss this issue with you or their GP. Many men feel isolated and worthless, and have no self-esteem at all. So summon up some courage to go to your doctor. He or she will have seen it all before and will get you on the road to recovery. You can ask for a referral to an ED clinic at the local hospital – not all doctors are qualified to talk about ED problems. Try and attend with your partner.

I feel so sorry for my partner who just can't get an erection any more. It is stressing him out. Is there anything I can do to reduce the strain on him?

The sexual response is associated with an excitement phase. However, the way the blood vessels react in order to get more blood in to the genitals (the penis in the man, the vulva and clitoris in the woman) is for those blood vessels to relax and dilate. Any sort of pressure, anxiety or stress on either partner in a sexual relationship may lead to these blood vessels staying constricted and causing a lack of either engorgement or vulval and clitoral swelling. Many myths surround sex and sexuality and, if your partner is experiencing any of these, then he needs to talk to someone about them, either his GP, practice nurse or counsellor, but one of the best people for him to talk to is you. One way of reducing sexual tension in a relationship is to ignore these myths and concentrate on what is good for the two of you. Sex doesn't have to last for any given length of time nor be of any definite frequency or type, but needs to be right for the people in that relationship.

You can reduce the stress of having sex by communication, positive feedback, and not making any disparaging remarks about a partner's prior failure. Many men suffer from performance anxiety, which is where they think an erection will fail, and then it does and further reinforces this very significant psychological problem. One way you can help him overcome this problem would be to reassure him that sexual satisfaction can be achieved without the need for penetration and therefore for an erection. You can help him by praising his sexual successes, playing down any failures and reassuring him that you can both be sexually satisfied without penetration. If your partner is wary of sex without penetration, tell him that foreplay and even oral sex can be very satisfying.

I have heard that impotence sufferers have an increased risk of prostate cancer. Is this true?

This question has several aspects. Firstly, a proportion of men who have prostate cancer also have ED. This is because the majority of men with both of these problems are in the age group over 50 years (the age when prostate cancer and impotence become more common), but there is no evidence that having ED itself causes prostate cancer. The other side of this is 'Does prostate cancer cause ED?' This is the case in only very few people, where the prostate cancer spreads outside of the prostate gland itself to affect the surrounding nerves. Thirdly, treatment

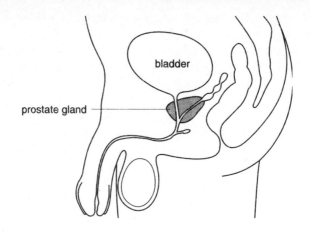

Figure 1.2 Position of prostate gland.

for prostate cancer *can* cause ED. This is particularly true if the cancer had spread and the surgeon has had to take away the nerves lying next to the prostate (Figure 1.2). This is the so-called 'non-nerve sparing prostatectomy' (see Chapter 9). Before any procedure for prostate cancer, your surgeon will discuss with you the likelihood of you having ED after your operation.

Can having an erection for too long be bad for you?

Only in very exceptional circumstances. After ejaculation, the blood normally drains away from the penis. If this does not happen and the erection is prolonged for 4 hours or more, you need to seek medical help immediately. The medical term for this problem is *priapism*, named after the Greek god Priapus who had an everlasting erection! We talk more about this in Chapter 2.

What can I do if I get an erection but it doesn't last?

This is a very common problem for men with sexual dysfunction. The first important issue here is whether you lose your erection because of rapid ejaculation (where you come too quickly), or whether you lose it before ejaculation or before penetration has taken place, or just as you are about to insert your penis into your partner's vagina – this might be due to psychological problems, which are discussed in the section *All in the mind?* in Chapter 2. If you lose the erection before ejaculation, then the modern thinking is that there is insufficient blood in the penis to sustain your erection. This thinking is at odds with a previous idea that a 'venous leakage' has occurred (meaning that blood was leaking from the veins). Urological surgeons attempted to repair this 'venous leakage' by surgery, but this proved to be unsuccessful in the long term. Modern treatment is to give drugs that will get more blood coming in to the penis. These drugs are discussed in Chapters 6 and 7 and can be either given by mouth or inserted directly in to the penis.

I am not ejaculating as much sperm as I used to. Why?

We need to find out here whether you mean the amount of fluid ejaculated or the numbers of sperm inside the fluid. 'Semen' has two main components – sperm (or seed), which originates in the

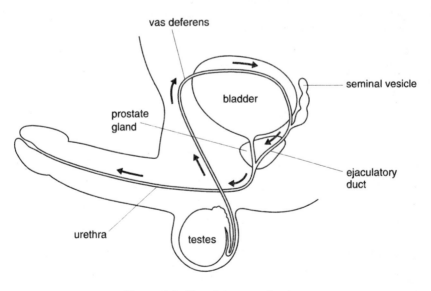

Figure 1.3 Ejaculatory mechanism.

testicles, and 'seminal fluid', which originates in the seminal vesicles and the prostate gland. The problem of decreased ejaculate is either due to less production or to a problem in the ejaculatory mechanism. A hormone called testosterone controls production. It is very common as men get older for their levels of testosterone to decrease, and therefore the amount of ejaculate to decrease also. This is only a significant problem if it is associated with male infertility, i.e. the amount of sperm or seed inside the fluid decreases to an extent where a man cannot fertilize his partner.

The second problem involving the ejaculatory mechanism (Figure 1.3) is relatively rare. Part of the ejaculatory process is the closure of the bladder neck. This closure is controlled by the nervous system. Therefore diseases such as diabetes or other neurological problems, or spinal cord injury, can all affect the nerves that control this mechanism, and can cause retrograde ejaculation, where semen is ejaculated up into the bladder rather than out through the penis. The same damage to the bladder neck mechanism can be caused by pelvic surgery and particularly surgery to either the bladder neck or the prostate gland.

Very rarely, you might not have any ejaculation fluid at all. This is most commonly caused by psychological factors such as a fear of getting your partner pregnant, but it can also very rarely be due to surgery (we discuss this further in Chapter 10). Again, do visit your doctor. He will be able to find out exactly what you mean and what the best course of action for you, and possibly your partner, will be, especially if you fear that you might be infertile.

Up until recently my erections have been good, with initial use of Viagra, but now I have noticed that I am ejaculating too quickly. This is causing me more distress than the impotence. I have never suffered from this before. My partner now doesn't want to have sex, as she finds it frustrating when I ejaculate within seconds of having penetrative sex. What can I do?

Ejaculating too quickly is called rapid ejaculation (RE). Your RE is probably due to anxiety or fear of losing the erection. When men start to suffer from ED, they find that their erections gradually become weaker, or they lose their erections quicker. So they start to reduce the amount of foreplay and have penetrative sex quicker, and hence ejaculate quicker, before they lose the erection altogether, to try and overcome the problem. This is a common problem for men when they haven't previously been able to get an erection and now can. We talk more about RE in Chapter 11.

I seem to lose my erection when I put on a condom. I like to practise safe sex and would want to continue to use one. Have I got ED?

It is very probable that you haven't got ED. Quite often, when you put on a condom, it is invariably tight, gets stuck after passing over the head of the penis, especially if you are uncircumcised, and consequently you put it on clumsily resulting in a loss of erection. What you are actually doing is pushing the blood back down from your penis into your body. Try the following and see if these tips help:

- Use K-Y Jelly or something similar while your penis is erect.

- Ensure that your fingernails are short.

- Open the condom packet.

- Insert your thumbs into the condom and use your forefingers to roll the condom down until it is open enough to cover the head of your penis and the start of the shaft.

- Release the condom onto the shaft (extracting your thumbs) and roll it over the penis down to the base.

2

Causes of sexual dysfunction

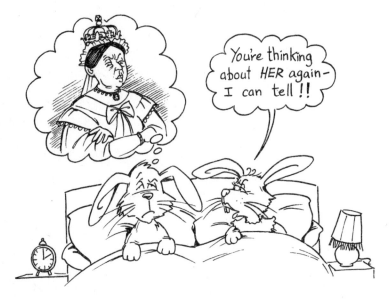

Erections are all about getting blood into the penis. Erections are funny things because they start in the mind and finish in the penis! Therefore anything that disturbs the mental processes associated with sexual excitation can affect the ability to gain a satisfactory penile erection. Equally diseases that affect the nerves and the blood vessels in the penis and throughout the body can also be associated with problems in gaining an erection. One of the most common misconceptions about sexual dysfunction is the role that hormones play. Many men think or want to believe that erectile failure is due to a hormonal imbalance, in particular a lack of testosterone. All these issues are discussed in this chapter.

Role of hormones

I have problems with getting a good erection. Is it something to do with my hormones?

While it is true that testosterone (the male hormone) decreases with age, there is no direct link between testosterone and the ability to gain an erection. Castrated men, such as eunuchs, can still have sexual activity, as was demonstrated in the harems of central Asia – they were still able to have sex with women, despite having had their testicles surgically removed. There is no evidence that treating men who have erectile failure with hormone replacement resolves any of these problems.

However, testosterone as the main male hormone does have an important role in sexual response. A lack of testosterone can show itself in several ways:

- a low sexual drive (called in the medical world 'libido'), although in the vast majority of adult men this is caused by psychological rather than hormonal factors;
- a decrease in body hair, e.g. a lack of facial, axillary (armpit) and pubic hair (covering sexual areas);
- decreased testicular size.

There is a debate amongst doctors as to whether a testosterone level test should be made as part of an examination for erectile failure. However, most doctors feel that this test is unnecessary unless there are signs, such as a decrease in body hair, which would suggest a low testosterone level. In your case you are probably aware of any of these signs and, if you think that you might have a low level, it would be worth discussing the problem with your doctor. If you have a badly damaged spine, a blood test of the testosterone level may be normal, but it will be soaked up by the spine and not reach the genitals.

Abnormalities with the thyroid gland can also lead to sexual problems. Thyroid disease in men can cause a variety of sexual problems, including problems with erection and problems with ejaculation. Having too much of the thyroid hormones (hyperthyroidism) causes the body to speed up and will be associated with rapid ejaculation. Having not enough of the thyroid hormones (hypothyroidism) will cause the body to slow down and both men and women will tend to have problems reaching orgasm (such as delayed ejaculation).

I am in my late 50s. I was so worried about not having sex any more that I had a hormone test done, but my testosterone levels were normal. Do I just put it down to age?

Studies made throughout the world have been remarkably consistent. They show that 50% of men aged 50 years and older will have some degree of ED and 10% will have no erections at all. These percentages rise as men get older.

As you get older, ED can occur because of 'atherosclerosis', which is a hardening of the blood vessels and arteries, the major cause of men having high blood pressure, heart attacks and strokes. It can cause equal problems in the blood vessels involved with erections. We talk about how this can be helped later on in this chapter.

However, the key message is that age in itself should not be a barrier to having a good sex life. You and your partner should be able to stay sexually active for as long as you both want to do so. Therefore, it is very important for everyone to realize that age should not be a barrier to treatment for sexual dysfunction, and with help you should get your sex life back.

So, if it's not due to hormones and not just due to my age, what does cause my erections to fail?

As we said at the beginning of this chapter, erections are important things because they start in the mind and finish in the penis. Therefore, pretty much anything affecting either the thought processes or the blood vessels or nerves can affect your ability to have an erection. The causes that relate to the thought processes are called 'psychological' (psychogenic – meaning 'originating in the brain') and those relating to the blood vessels and nerves 'physical' (organic), but most men will have a combination of both psychogenic and organic causes and hence the wide variety of treatments aimed at both causes individually can be applied to virtually every man with ED. Every time a man suffers from erection failure, regardless of reason, then he can start to develop 'performance anxiety'.

All in the mind?

I can't seem to get hard with my wife – we've been married for 30 years – so I feel I have a problem, but I often get an erection at work! I feel very guilty about this and can't discuss it with my wife. What should I do?

Most men who suffer from ED have mixed causes for erection failure, both physical and psychological. Every time a man suffers from erection failure, regardless of reason, then he can start to develop 'performance anxiety'. If you can get an erection when you:

- masturbate
- wake up
- see something that arouses you, or
- are with a non-regular partner

but can't get aroused when you want to or lose a strong erection when you start to have penetrative sex, then this may be due to psychological causes rather than physical. ED from psychogenic causes is found in about 20% of cases, and is particularly common in younger men with ED (about 70% of cases under 35 years).

If you can never get an erection or can only get a semi-erection when you masturbate or have foreplay, and it doesn't matter what the situation is, then your ED is probably physical.

If your erections gradually got worse, rather than suddenly, then this also could be physical, unless something has suddenly happened to affect your health, e.g. heart attack, car accident, stroke or pelvic surgery. You might have changed medications or started on a new one, and find you lose your ability to have an erection quickly – this could be due to the medication itself.

The best way of establishing if your erection failure is due to physical causes or if it's 'all in your mind' is to go to your GP for further assessment.

I had a very strict upbringing and wasn't allowed to see a girl until I was 21. I find it very difficult to hold down any relationship now. Could this be causing my problems in the bed department?

There are lots of psychological causes of erection problems:

- those that predispose a man (or make him susceptible) to have ED;
- those that precipitate (bring on) ED;
- those that, once a man has ED, make sure he always has it (maintaining factors).

The box on pages 19–20 explains these in more detail.

Although many symptoms that people discuss with their doctors seem to be caused by psychological problems, the vast majority of men have both psychological and physical problems going on at the same time. Don't be embarrassed about talking over your worries – the doctor is there to help you.

I don't seem to fit into any real pattern that you are talking about, but I can't make love to my partner. If it is a psychological problem, is there anything else I could look for?

Yes, ED is more likely to be 'all in your mind' if:

- it occurs in some social circumstances but not in others (what doctors and nurses call 'situational'), or with some partners and not others;
- you are able to gain and maintain an erection during masturbation, but not in a sexual relationship;
- you find that you have firm erections at other times during the day, but not in a sexually stimulating environment;

- you have other psychological problems, such as marked stress, anxiety or depression.

However, over the last few years, as the physical causes and the role that heart disease plays in ED have been better understood, it is now thought that the vast majority of men with ED have a combination of physical and psychological factors. Clearly, there will be some people at one end of the spectrum and

---

Psychological causes of ED

Predisposing factors
- *Restricted upbringing.* A 'Victorian'-type upbringing might lead to repression of sexuality associated with feelings of guilt. Similar effects can be brought about by religious or cultural pressures.
- *Traumatic sexual experience.* Sexual abuse as a child or to humiliation by a partner in an early sexual encounter can both lead to ED.
- *Poor sexual education.* Lack of adequate sex education can lead to unrealistic expectations by either partner.
- *Disturbed family relationships.* If you were overly fond of somebody in your family or even had a desire to have sex with your mother or father (called the Oedipus complex), then you could well suffer with problems with intercourse now.
- *Lifestyle problems.* Men who are too stressed in their daily life from work and financial worries often cannot 'perform'.
- *Personality type.* Some personality types seem to be more prone to ED than others.

Precipitating factors
- *Ageing.* With increasing age, men take longer to get aroused. Accordingly, more time and foreplay is needed to attain a rigid penis. If you don't give each other time, you might not be aroused enough to get a good erection.

Psychological causes of ED (continued)

- *Infidelity.* Infidelity and guilt bring on failure in either your relationship with your long-term partner, or the illicit one (or both).
- *Unreasonable expectations.* The performance expectation of either partner can sometimes be unreasonably high, and remember that men and women have differing peaks of arousal during the month.
- *Depression and anxiety.* Both depression and anxiety can precipitate ED, although the effects are not uniform from person to person. It is important to remember that many antidepressant and antihypertension medications can also cause ED. (See the section on **Depression and stress** in Chapter 3.)
- *Loss of partner.* The so-called 'widower's syndrome' can result from the death of your partner, divorce or separation, and can lead to a complete loss of erections for some time.

Maintaining factors

- *Performance anxiety.* Prior failure leads to increased levels of anxiety, and this inhibits sexual performance. This appears to be one of the most important features of psychological ED.
- *Diminished attraction for one's partner.* This can happen in any relationship and suggests that therapy might not be successful, but counselling might well help.
- *Poor communication within a relationship.* If you don't discuss your sexual problems with your partner, things will probably not get better. Again, counselling and learning to talk about problems will help.
- *Fear of intimacy.* This is often associated with family upbringing.
- *Poor sexual education.* Inadequate education can lead to so-called 'sexual myths' being perpetuated, which not only predispose to, but can also maintain sexual dysfunction.
- *Poor general relationship.* If your relationship is a poor one, then you may have problems recovering sexual function within that relationship, but counselling can help here, if you are both willing to try it.

some at the other. So, if most men have a combination of factors causing their dysfunction, then most should be offered treatment with both drugs and psychosexual counselling. You can opt for one or other of these treatments, or a combination of both, after you have been given the pros and cons of each by the healthcare professional assessing you. See also Chapters 5–9 on various different types of treatments available.

Physical causes

Atherosclerosis

I am in my 60s and have been diagnosed with athero- sclerosis. I have real problems sustaining any real sex with my wife. Has my diagnosis anything to do with it?

Atherosclerosis is a hardening of the arteries, which can lead to high blood pressure or cause a reduction in blood supply to the heart (ischaemia) and this causes chest pain (called angina).

Just as the arteries in the heart harden, then the arteries in the penis can harden. Atherosclerosis causes about half of all the cases of ED in men over 50 years of age. The hardening of the arteries reduces the circulation to the penis, and when a man gets aroused his penis is unable to cope with the surge of blood necessary to get an erect penis.

Erections are all about getting blood into the penis. Any disease that is bad for the blood vessels and circulation will also be bad for erections. These include diseases such as diabetes, high blood pressure and high levels of cholesterol. Smoking can also cause problems with circulation. Doctors now know that erection problems may indicate blood vessel disease, and therefore, if you have erection problems, you should first see a doctor rather than seek cures just for your sexual problem, in order to have your overall health assessed. There are lots of treatments that sort the problem out.

The opening up of these blood vessels is under the control of the nervous system as are many sensations causing erections, such as touch. Therefore the second important element is an intact nervous system. Erections begin when the brain receives sexually stimulating impulses, which then trigger a release of chemicals, which begin a sexual response. There are many causes for an interruption to this flow of events, both psychological (mentioned above) and physical (such as multiple sclerosis or diabetes). Clearly anything that leads to depression, anxiety or stress can affect a person's ability to respond sexually.

Because many cases of impotence are due to reduced blood flow from blocked arteries, it is important to maintain good general health by following the same lifestyle suggestions for those who face an increased risk for heart disease. The box below shows some of these suggestions.

What can I do to prevent ED in the future?

- Quit smoking, if you smoke.
- Moderate your alcohol intake.
- Have a good balanced diet, which includes a lot of fresh fruits and vegetables, whole grains and fibre, and which is low in saturated fats and sodium.
- Ensure that your diet includes vitamin E and possibly zinc (this is probably sound advice but there is no research to prove it).
- Take regular exercise.
- If you stay sexually active, this can help prevent impotence. If you have frequent erections, blood flow to the penis will be stimulated.
- Change or reduce medications known to affect erections. Do not stop taking your medication until you have spoken to your GP first.
- Control your stress level.
- Make time for yourself and your partner.
- Try visual and 'fantasy' stimulation.

Stress

I get very stressed by my job as an editor, and I know that this is affecting my sex life (and my drinking). Could a change in my lifestyle improve my sexual performance?

There are numerous reasons why lifestyle impacts on sexual function. Firstly, sexual relationships need time and energy put in to them. If you and your partner are each working 70–80 hours per week and see each other only intermittently, or only when you are very tired, then this will have a negative impact on both your desire and ability to have sex. Secondly, sex does require physical exertion and, if minimal exertion leads you to become extremely breathless or have chest pain, then this will affect your ability to function sexually. Thirdly, getting aroused depends on the ability to relax and succumb to sexual stimuli. If you are stressed and anxious about work or money for instance, then you will not be affected by sexual stimuli and thus you may find it difficult to become sexually aroused. Fourthly, if your lifestyle involves the use of excess social drugs or alcohol, you will also find it more difficult to get aroused.

Spinal cord injuries and the central nervous system

ED is a common problem in men who suffer from central nervous system and/or spinal cord disorders. Men who suffer from central nervous system disorders such as multiple sclerosis, Parkinson's disease, temporal lobe epilepsy or Alzheimer's disease have an increased risk of suffering from impotence, particularly from the therapy that they are receiving. Men suffering from spinal cord disorders caused by spinal cord injury (SCI), spina bifida, spinal cord compression, or who have had surgical or radiation injury to pelvic nerves, pelvic fracture injury or peripheral neuropathy have a high risk factor of suffering from ED.

I have damaged my spinal cord through falling off a ladder. Whilst in hospital I was told that my back injury might cause me to be impotent. Is this true?

How your erections are affected will depend on the severity, type of injury and time since you damaged your spinal cord. If your spinal cord injury has been defined as incomplete, then you are at less risk of suffering from impotence. If you have damaged the lower part of your spinal cord then you have a higher risk of impotence but, if you damaged your spine higher up, then usually men have the ability to achieve an erection.

Impotence in men who have received a spinal cord injury may only be short term. It may take a year for their erections to recover. You may or may not be able to achieve an erection in the future but, if you are not able to, there is a vast amount of therapies available that will help you obtain and maintain an erection.

Since damaging my back my erections haven't been as strong as before the accident. Is this common?

Yes, this is possible. Many men complain about having poorer quality erections after having a spinal cord injury. It is advisable that you go and seek help and information from your GP, or that your GP refers you, if he or she doesn't feel appropriately trained in assessing your erection problems, as there are numerous treatments available on prescription that will help improve your erections. Referral can be to a sex therapist, ED specialists at hospitals, or to an orthopaedic surgeon.

Since having a car accident I am unable to get a spontaneous erection but when I masturbate I can get a fairly strong erection that I am able to have sex with. Why is this?

That is because there are two types of erections, 'psychogenic erections' and 'reflexogenic erections'.

Psychogenic erections result when messages are passed down the spinal cord from the brain to the sacral or genital area.

Psychogenic erections are a result of having sexual thoughts, or by being aroused by your senses, seeing and hearing things that arouse you. This is dependent on the level and completeness of the injury to the spinal cord; therefore men with SCI may or may not experience psychogenic erections. In men with lower level injuries, research has shown that up to 83% with incomplete lower level injuries had psychogenic erections and up to 26% of men with complete lesions have psychogenic erections. In men with incomplete upper level injuries, up to 25% can achieve psychogenic erections.

Reflexogenic erections are controlled by a reflex arc between the genital area and the spinal cord. Therefore reflexogenic erections are a result from direct stimulation of the genital area, either by self-masturbation or by your partner. Current research has shown that 98% of men who have suffered from upper level spinal injuries are able to have reflexogenic erections and up to 93% of men with complete upper level injuries have reflexogenic erections.

Other trauma

I do a lot of cycling, can this be responsible for my poor erections?

Cycling can be responsible for genital discomfort in up to 90% of cyclists and could lead to ED. This is because the classically designed bicycle seat, after prolonged use, leads to compression of the perineal nerves – these are the nerves around the penis, anus and buttocks, and the tops of the thighs, leading to loss of sensation in that area affecting the ability of the blood vessels to relax and allow sufficient blood into the area for penile or vulval engorgement. Standing up on the pedals every 10 minutes and sitting as upright as possible may help.

I damaged my hip skiing last year. Could an accident be the cause of impotence?

Trauma to the pelvis that has disrupted the blood vessels or nerves supplying the genitals can lead to sexual dysfunction. However, trauma related to the hip itself should not cause any damage. If there is any ongoing pain or disability in the area, then this might distract you during sex. Your doctor can give you pain-relieving treatment, but it would be best to mention why you need it.

My friend had to go into hospital recently because he says he fractured his penis – he didn't say how he did it! I have never heard of this before – was he telling me the truth?

Yes it is possible, particularly from very vigorous lovemaking. It is a very painful accident caused by tearing of the fibrous tissues in the penis. Not a laughing matter!

Prolonged erections

My friends laugh because I get prolonged erections. It's embarrassing and often painful. What are these caused by and what can be done?

Prolonged erections are called priapism (see Chapter 1). These are often caused by the actual treatment for ED, such as injections into the penis that work too well, but they can, rarely, be the result of certain medical conditions, such as sickle cell disease, or the side effects of antidepressants such as fluoxetine (Prozac), sertraline (Lustral), or other drugs used to treat rapid ejaculation.

Lifestyle

I have trouble getting an erection these days. I do drink more than I used to. Would giving up alcohol help? I like drinking and find it a great comfort.

Excess alcohol intake is associated with 'brewer's droop' where you find it difficult to have sex because your penis refuses to get hard! A small amount of alcohol is a stimulant and some people find it facilitates a sexual encounter. However, a much greater amount of alcohol will act as a depressant and make an individual less coherent and sleepier, thus making it more difficult to gain a penile erection. In the majority of times when ED is caused by alcohol, it is reversible – you just need to stop drinking. The only way of knowing if your ED has been caused by the alcohol is by stopping the alcohol. Even if the alcohol hasn't caused the erectile problems, then you will need to reduce your alcohol intake to be able to get the best results out of ED treatment. Reduce your alcohol – your liver will thank you for it.

'Iatrogenic' causes

My doctor has said that my failure in the bedroom depart-ment is due to surgery that I had or my pills. Is this true?

ED is sometimes thought to have been caused by medical care ('iatrogenic' causes). This can include ED:

- following surgery to the prostate
- following radiotherapy for prostate cancer,
- being drug related, e.g. associated with tablets to control blood pressure.

If you develop impotence after starting tablets for high blood pressure, see your doctor straight away. Do not stop them before going to see your doctor, but there are alternatives available with fewer side effects.

Venous leakage

The doctor said my ED is caused by venous leakage. What is that?

Venous leakage was thought previously to be a cause of erectile dysfunction by many doctors, the theory being that, if you could obtain an erection, but could not maintain it, then this could be due to the blood flowing back out of your penis through your veins – a venous leak. This leak would reduce the amount of blood in the penis and so reduce its firmness. The diagnosis has gone out of favour as, although there is a reasonably simple operation to surgically stop these leaking veins, the results of this surgery has been very disappointing as regards long-term cures for ED.

You might wish to try other forms of treatment first, for example Viagra, Uprima or other oral ED therapies (see Chapter 7 on *Medical oral treatments*), or vacuum therapy devices (see Chapter 9).

3
Sexual dysfunction and other conditions

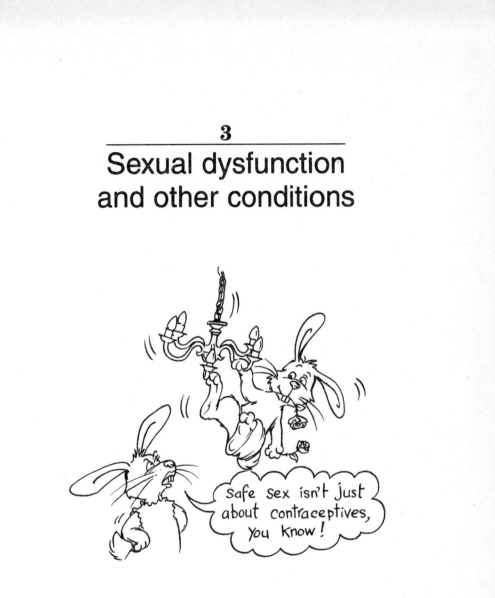

As erections are all about getting blood into the penis and the blood vessels (arteries and veins) are under the control of the nervous system, any condition that affects the nervous system can also affect erections. We discuss here some of those conditions.

Multiple sclerosis

As a relatively young man with MS, I am sure that I am having some sexual problems that I reckon are due to the MS. Do you think that's likely? Do other men with MS have sexual problems?

Of course sexual problems can take many forms, and almost all of them can affect anybody, with or without MS. As you may be aware, it is quite difficult to obtain accurate statistics about the relative sexual problems of people with and without MS. Nevertheless, it does appear that sexual problems of several kinds do seem to be more likely amongst men with MS. Studies have shown that over 70% of men under 50 with mild MS experience problems in their sexual abilities compared with 20% of non-MS people, and 80% have problems with erections or ejaculation. We know that most men with MS don't have sexual intercourse so frequently as men without MS, and their interest in or satisfaction with intercourse is also lower. Many men with MS report problems with orgasm (coming) – often associated with rapid or retarded ejaculation – problems with fatigue, and lower levels of masturbation.

These sexual problems appear to be closely related to problems with bladder or bowel dysfunction, and with spasticity (stiffness) in the legs. However, there are three particular kinds of sexual dysfunction often associated with MS:

- Some problems are directly related to changes in the nerve pathways damaged by the MS – and this is often called **primary sexual dysfunction**.
- Problems caused by MS affecting other parts of the body, or body systems, indirectly affecting sexual performance, are called **secondary sexual dysfunction**.
- Further problems may be related to personal, social or cultural issues that make sexual activity more difficult – often called **tertiary sexual dysfunction**.

All three dysfunctions probably occur either at the same time or at different times, and they might influence each other. For example, fears about future sexual performance (a tertiary dysfunction), partly derived from occasional or frequent erectile difficulties (often a primary dysfunction), may create further difficulties, compounded by mobility problems or fatigue (secondary dysfunctions). Disentangling the relationship between all these factors requires careful analysis and then careful management. It can be done so you should be able to have a very satisfying sex life. With modern treatments available, it is worth asking your doctor for help.

With my MS I'm really having a difficulty 'performing' sexually. Most of the time I can't get an erection. What's the problem?

At a 'mechanical' level you might not get an erection either because of problems in the blood supply to your penis or problems in the control of erections and ejaculation by your nervous system, and this is much more likely in MS.

Managing erectile problems in principle means focusing on three sets of possible problems:

- those in the nervous system;
- those associated with the blood supply system, and
- those arising from psychological and related issues.

At present there are no means of restoring already damaged nervous system pathways, so you will be helped best by stimulation of the blood supply and resolving psychological problems. As mentioned in the previous question, there are modern treatments available to help with the last two problems (see the following chapters on treatment).

I really don't feel like having sex any more. Is this the result of the MS? I am worried that my relationship with my partner is now deteriorating badly as a result. What can I do?

It is often difficult to disentangle the various changes occurring as a result of MS from other factors. Sometimes symptoms like depression or fatigue, which are indirect (or secondary) symptoms of MS, may play as large a part, in the way that you feel sexually, as primary neurological damage does. If such symptoms are treated successfully, then your sexual drive (often called your *libido*) may increase.

If the main cause of your decreasing sexual drive lies in primary neurological damage, then this is harder to deal with directly. You and your partner could perhaps consider other means of having a sensual set of experiences, without you feeling the immediate pressure for sexual intercourse – other parts of your body may be more erotically sensitive. With gentle mutual touch and exploration you may find, as many other couples have done both with and without MS, that you can introduce a new sensual and loving element into your relationship. Make time to enjoy the experiences with each other without feeling hurried or under pressure. Most relationships involve planning – it is just that with MS a little more planning is required.

The stiffness in my legs proved to be a big problem when I tried to have sexual intercourse recently with my girlfriend. Is there any advice you can offer me about this?

The effect of unexpected spasms in your legs, or elsewhere, during sexual activity, can be very disconcerting. The important thing is to check with your doctor that the general control of your stiffness (spasticity) is as good as it can be. The normal approach is to try and keep your muscles as well toned as possible through regular exercises and to use appropriate drugs, such as baclofen, as necessary to give additional control.

There are also certain positions for sexual activity that appear to make the muscular spasms less likely, although it is important that you explore other possibilities than those mentioned below, for you may find a position that suits you both very well, which is not described here. If you have difficulty with spasms or rigidity in your legs, then sitting in an appropriate chair (without arms) would allow your partner to sit on your penis, either facing you or with her back to you.

Fatigue is my major problem when it comes to sex. I just don't feel I have the energy. What can I do?

Many people with MS find that fatigue is a problem with a great many of their activities, owing to its often unpredictable nature. As with other symptoms associated with MS, it is important to discuss this with your doctor who will assess the best means of managing it. There are one or two drugs that may help (for example amantadine or pemoline), which can be taken a few minutes before sexual activity. Currently the best help is through various appropriate lifestyle changes.

One obvious way forward is to consider at what times you feel least tired. Although this may not necessarily be the time when you feel that you should be having sex – such as in the morning, or during the day, rather than at a more conventional time – you may be less tired and enjoy it more. Rather than thinking of sexual intercourse as the major element, you could agree with your partner to engage in some other less energetic sexual activities – such as gentle stroking or foreplay – that you could participate in more frequently. As with so many other aspects of living with MS, it is a question of finding ways to adapt to the situation through experimentation.

I feel I am unusual as someone with MS who is gay. Almost all the advice I read about sexuality and MS implies that people are heterosexual and are in opposite sex partnerships. Is there any recognition of the problems that people like me face?

You are quite right that, until recently, it has not been recognized at all that some people with MS are gay. Even in the increasing material that is being written about sexuality and disabled people, the particular problems of being gay are often not covered. According to national surveys, perhaps 1 in 10 people with MS is gay, so there may be many people with MS who feel as you do.

The MS Society has recently established a lesbian and gay group. Details can be obtained from the national MS Society. For disabled and non-disabled lesbian and bisexual women, it would also be worth contacting SPOD (the association to aid the sexual and personal relationships of people with a disability) for further information and advice. (All these addresses can be found in Appendix 1.)

I have MS and am young and single. Most of the information available on sexuality seems to be for people who are in long-term relationships with another person. Can you give me any advice?

Yes, it is often assumed that the majority of the population both with and without MS is already in a stable, usually married, long-term relationship. In fact, most of the adult population with or without MS, including those who have been divorced or whose relationships have broken down, are single; there are an increasing number of single parents, and those whose partner has died. We live in a society where people are in many different forms of relationships. Gradually the information available for people with MS is reflecting this situation, and it is not very different from advice anyone needs.

Advice regarding sex and sexuality in young people with MS really depends on your individual problem. In general, the same advice will hold regardless of age, in that sex is all about communicating your fears and anxieties to a new sexual partner. Despite this potentially being very frightening, it will, in the vast majority of cases, help you. Just talking to the person with whom you want sex, or to a third party, such as a counsellor, will be beneficial. Many of the questions and answers here should cover any problems that you have. Talk to your doctor who oversees your MS about your problems – if he or she is not able to help or advise you, you will be referred to a specialist.

Parkinson's disease

Does Parkinson's cause impotence? My husband has become impotent at the age of 39, four years after being diagnosed.

Yes. ED is common in many diseases that affect the central nervous system, such as Parkinson's, MS and motor neurone disease. There are treatments that will help your husband overcome the complications and these are discussed in later chapters. He might need your help in giving some of the treatments. Ask your GP to refer him to a specialist. It would be worth getting in touch with the Parkinson's Disease Society (address in Appendix 1) as they offer advice by telephone, or in leaflets or on their website.

There is a pamphlet called *Parkinson's disease and sex* (available from the Parkinson's Disease Society – details in Appendix 1), which has a straightforward discussion of the nature of sexual function and sexual problems, as well as information gathered together from people with Parkinson's. Stress, anxiety and depression seemed to be more important causes of problems than anything directly related to the disease, and counselling can usually help here.

Heart disease and high blood pressure

I have high blood pressure for which I am taking tablets. I am having problems with getting an erection. What advice can you give me?

There are several aspects to this question. Firstly, taking any medication for high blood pressure does not stop a man using treatments for his ED, including all the licensed therapies both taken orally and used directly on the penis (see later chapters on treatment).

The second issue is that some people think that their medication given for high blood pressure (antihypertensive treatment) has caused their ED. You might have noticed this only when the antihypertensive treatment was started. The real problem, however, lies in the underlying disease process, which has narrowed your blood vessels and hence caused your blood pressure to rise, and stop the blood flowing to the penis. **It is very important, if your doctor has put you onto antihypertensive medication, not to stop it if ED follows, but to return to your doctor and discuss this issue with him**. The antihypertensive medication will protect your heart from a heart attack, and your brain from stroke. Your doctor can easily prescribe another medication to control your blood pressure and this could help your ED. It is, however, true that some of the older drugs treating high blood pressure do cause more problems than some of the newer drugs. So your doctor may decide to change your treatment for high blood pressure to see if one medication can control both your blood pressure and the erectile problems.

I have had a heart transplant. Should I be having sex at all?

As long as you have resumed normal daily activity, then there is no reason why you should not resume sexual activity. However, remember that, if you still need your nitrate spray, then you cannot be treated with Viagra, Cialis or Levitra (see Chapter 7), but there are other choices open to you.

I have been diagnosed with heart disease. I am worried that I won't be able to have treatment for my sexual problems. Will the doctor give me any medication?

The answer to this question depends on the severity of the disease. If you have controlled hypertension, mild heart valve disease, mild stable angina or successful revascularization of your heart, your GP will be able to manage your ED. If you have had a recent heart attack or stroke (i.e. within the last 6 weeks), or you have a heart murmur of unknown cause or moderate stable angina, then *specialist* evaluation is recommended, with an exercise test for angina and an echocardiograph for the murmur. If, however, you have been diagnosed with 'unstable' or 'refractory angina', uncontrolled hypertension, recent myocardial infarction or stroke (i.e. within the last 14 days), high-risk arrhythmia or hypertrophic cardiomyopathy, then treatment for your ED should be delayed until your heart condition has been stabilized. So take heart – your doctor can help!

Is there a relationship between heart disease and ED?

Erections are all about getting blood into the penis and so any condition that affects the blood vessels will be related to ED. In people with untreated hypertension, 17% have ED; in those who are diabetic, 30% have ED, but in those people who have had a previous heart attack, 44% will have ED.

Is casual sex more stressful to the heart than sex with a partner in a long-term relationship?

Yes, casual sex can be more stressful. Long-standing relationships, where people are comfortable with each other, should present no problem, but a casual encounter can lead to a greater heart rate rise. This is not harmful to a normal heart, but if coronary disease is present, problems could occur. There may be an age mismatch (e.g. older man, younger woman) and the environment unfamiliar (e.g. hotel room), or too much food and drink may have been consumed (and casual sex at an office party, for example, might follow). Playing 'away from home' can be more risky. If you are gay and have casual sex, then unprotected sex could also be stressful.

You sometimes hear horror stories of people dying while they are making love. Are these stories true?

You can die at any time and this includes during sex! The risk during sex is very low indeed and no higher than during other normal daily activities. It may be significant that, of those who die

or have a heart attack during sex, 80% are having extramarital sex
– so the advice is, beware!

I had a heart attack recently. How soon can I start making love again?

After a heart attack, provided that there were no complications,
sexual activity can be resumed in 2–3 weeks. Try using stairs,
walking or a treadmill test as your guide to see if you get short of
breath afterwards. Sex is a normal activity and not particularly
stressful for couples in a long-standing relationship and should be
enjoyed as much by those with heart disease as those without. As
you recover from a heart attack and return to normal activities,
you should be able to return to the normal activity of sex. The
amount of exercise associated with normal sexual activity is
equivalent to doing light housework!

Many men who have had a heart attack suffer from impotence;
if you do, talk to your doctor about it.

If you used oral therapy to help improve your erections before
your heart attack, then you need to talk to your doctor before
taking them again.

**I am in my early fifties and have had a heart attack. Am I
too old for sex?**

If you enjoyed sex before your heart attack there is no reason
why you shouldn't enjoy it again. Just listen to your body – if you
are getting breathless or noticing that you are having angina
pains, then stop until the symptoms have gone. You might need to
be a bit more imaginative with sexual positions than you were
before, but that will add to the pleasure. Age should never be a
barrier if you were previously sexually active – you should not be
afraid of resuming normal relations.

Men who have had a heart attack sometimes take longer
getting an erection and partners may worry about whether it is
safe for you to have sex. Don't rush sex – take your time, enjoy
the foreplay and the courtship.

I had heart surgery three weeks ago. My wife is keen to make love again. Can I resume lovemaking safely?

You can resume as soon as you feel able. If you get chest wall pain, particularly if you are positioned underneath your wife, then mutual foreplay without full sex can be a satisfying alternative and may be a good way to restart sexual activity. Alternatively, try other positions, such as the side-to-side position, and experiment to find one that is comfortable for both of you.

If you have had angioplasty (surgery to your blood vessels), you can resume sex within 2–3 days, depending on whether your groin is bruised or painful.

As a useful guide, making love is equal to walking briskly (1 mile on the flat in 20 minutes), or going up and down two flights of household stairs (about 12 steps in each flight) in about 10 seconds per flight. If no pain or undue breathlessness occurs, then sex should be symptom-free. If angina does occur during one of these tests, repeat it again after you have taken nitrate tablets under your tongue (sublingually) or by spray. If these drugs are effective, they can be taken before sex. Indeed, as a side effect, there is some evidence that nitrates improve sexual pleasure. Nitrates should not be used if Viagra, Levitra or Cialis have been taken (see Chapter 7 on *Medical oral treatments*).

My partner recently had heart surgery but has been given the all clear. Are some positions during lovemaking dangerous?

No, as long as you are sensible and don't try too many strenuous positions! Different sexual positions do not seem to lead to any excess stress on the heart. What does lead to more stress is having sex with a casual partner, so stay faithful if you are in a long-standing relationship; if you aren't in a long-term relationship, take things slowly.

Since I came back from hospital following a heart attack, I've had no interest in making love. It upsets my partner and frustrates her. What should I say to her?

Most people have sex as frequently as before a heart attack or surgery but others take it more easy. Some people are afraid that sex could damage the heart, and this fear spoils a previously enjoyable sex life. They are often influenced by the idea of what is called 'Hollywood sex', which is the movie portrayal of over-enthusiastic sex; in real life, sex isn't normally anything like as energetic, and the stress on the heart is therefore not so drastic.

Coming out of hospital can cause anxiety and depression and this could decrease your appetite for sex but, as your condition improves, your desire usually returns. Because you have a heart problem, you are now much more aware of the heart beating, whereas before it probably never worried you. Your heart beat will increase during lovemaking, but there is nothing to worry about: do the stair or walking test again (see earlier question) to reassure yourself.

If you are depressed after your heart attack or surgery, it usually lifts quickly, but a few people continue to feel depressed and this obviously reduces or removes your desire for sex. When you do make love, it is probably infrequent and not fulfilling. Don't accept this situation – you are not 'past it' – seek help from your doctor. Medication for depression, often for only a short time, is very effective and side effects are not usually a problem. We recommend you try cuddling and foreplay first to help you slowly return to a full sex life.

I have been diagnosed with angina. Will heart disease affect my sex drive?

No. There are too many people who believe in myths like this. Some think that their sex life is all over when they get to 50, when in fact you should be really enjoying life. In medical terms, you will be pleased to know that middle age extends now to 70 years! Once your symptoms have been dealt with, you should be able to resume lovemaking.

My wife and I have always had a vigorous and adventurous love life. Now I am worried that I might get angina while I am making love. Is this likely?

Angina could occur and is best treated with nitrates under your tongue or by using your GTN spray beforehand. Keep nitrates by the bedside, and take an extra spray or tablet if angina occurs during sex. Rest for 5–10 minutes, then resume if you wish to. If prolonged pain occurs, it could be a heart attack (and this is very unusual): if the pain persists after 30 minutes, seek medical help. If angina is severe enough to stop you having sex on a regular basis, ask your doctor for a full investigation and to be referred.

If you get breathless during sex, nitrates might help this but, if heart failure is the problem, your partner will need to adopt a more active role trying different positions. If you don't usually lie underneath, try this less stressful position or sit in a chair with your partner astride, facing you.

Remember, if you are using nitrates, you must not take Viagra, Cialis or Levitra.

To be honest, our love life wasn't up to much before the heart attack. Will it get worse?

If you were having sexual difficulties (such as lack of interest, poor satisfaction, or inability to sustain or develop an erection) before your heart problems, these may get worse. It is important to talk about these problems, either with the doctor or members of your cardiac rehabilitation team. Specific sexual counselling from trained counsellors will help.

I have heart failure and find that sex is too much effort. What can I do?

This is difficult because your heart's pumping action has been reduced. ACE inhibitors (for heart treatment) improve the heart's output and could help. Ask your doctor about them. Water pills (diuretics) may cause impotence as a side effect but you should not stop taking these. It may be possible to reduce the dosage or you could be given a different type, with fewer side effects. Unfortunately, if your breathing depends on taking diuretics, the dosage will not be reduced. Do **not** alter any of your medication unless advised to do so by your doctor, as this could have detrimental effects on the rest of your health and life.

Let your partner do most of the physical work. If you are finding that you can't get an erection, ask about injection treatment. This leads to an instant erection, which will last for the duration of intercourse. Viagra, Levitra or Cialis are alternatives. See Chapters 7 and 8 for more information on all these possibilities.

Heart failure can contribute to being unable to sustain a full sexual relationship, but cuddling, caressing, close contact and even foreplay will still enable you to enjoy a satisfying relationship.

I am taking medication for my heart problem. Can this affect my sex life? My wife says that I am not so interested as I used to be!

The most obvious side effect of some tablets is male impotence. Women can also become impotent (described as an inability to get an erect clitoris) but, because it is not so obvious, it is never mentioned or asked about. Medications that can cause impotence include the beta blockers and the diuretics. The statins (which reduce cholesterol) may, rarely, cause impotence. Women can become frigid and unable to have an orgasm, but this has not been clearly proved to be due to medication – it may be psychological and due to fear of damaging the heart, or there may be lubrication problems.

Whatever you do, don't stop your medication, as this may lead to more heart problems; equally, don't accept the situation. Talk to your doctor – this is not a time to be shy or 'British'. Ask your doctor whether the tablets might affect your sex life. When you collect medication from a pharmacy, it will come with patient information, so it is worthwhile reading this. The doctor will know what you are talking about. Changing medication or adjusting dosage often helps. If you are feeling depressed, antidepressants may correct the problem. However, if impotence or sexual dysfunction continues, it should be evaluated further. Specialist advice can be sought. Injection or MUSE therapy with prostaglandins can induce an erection very successfully if impotence persists and has not improved with a change in drugs. When you have been reviewed, then oral therapy may be a more appropriate way forward.

Since being on blood pressure pills, my husband is having a problem getting an erection. Is there a connection?

Yes. Blood pressure tablets can cause impotence in men but having hypertension (high blood pressure) carries a high risk even if you are not on treatment. So do not change or stop taking any medication that has been prescribed without talking to your doctor first. If this happens, your husband should tell his doctor because a change in medication could solve the problem. Impotence is more common with diuretics and beta blockers and less likely with ACE inhibitors, calcium antagonists and doxazosin (these are different types of blood pressure therapies).

Can you give me some advice in preparing for sex since my heart attack?

When heart disease has been diagnosed, it is important to follow the lifestyle changes that your GP will suggest. Doing more exercise and losing weight will help sexual ability also. Practical advice to minimize the stress on the heart during sex is as follows:

- Avoid sex within 2 hours of a bath or a heavy meal. Taking a shower instead of a bath and eating a light meal or snack instead of a heavy meal will be better.
- Keep the bedroom and sheets warm. You could invest in an electric blanket if it is cold.
- Don't make love if you are tired at the end of the day. Wait until the morning when you are refreshed and relaxed.
- Avoid caffeine, smoking or alcohol before or after sex. Alcohol raises expectations that you cannot fulfil and it

certainly does not enhance your sex life! However, one or two drinks may help to reduce anxiety.
- If you get angina, use your nitrate tablets before lovemaking.
- Don't rush into it – take your time.
- It is very important that your partner is well lubricated and using something like K-Y Jelly (available from pharmacies) or Sensilube (available from the Family Planning Association) may make insertion of the penis easier.

I am gay and have oral sex with my partner. Does oral or anal sex stress the heart?

Oral sex should not stress your heart, provided that both you and your partner are comfortable with it. There is some evidence that anal sex increases palpitations but this has not been proved in secure long-standing homosexual relationships.

I have resumed sex after my bypass and there are no problems, but I'm afraid that it might do some damage to the operation site. Is this possible?

Firstly, it is good to know that you have returned to a normal sexual relationship – we would like all people undergoing heart surgery such as yours to achieve this because it is safe and enjoyable. To answer your question directly: no, the operation site cannot be damaged, stitches will not be torn and nothing will fall apart! It is important to remember that sex should be an enjoyable fulfilling experience whether there is heart disease or not – people with heart disease can enjoy a sexual relationship whatever their age.

I have had some heart problems and my doctor talked about Kegel exercises for helping my ED. What exactly are these?

The Kegel exercise is a simple exercise commonly used by people who have urinary incontinence and by pregnant women (usually called pelvic floor exercises). It may also be helpful for men whose ED is caused by impaired blood circulation. The basic technique consists of tightening and releasing the pelvic muscle that controls urination. Since the muscle is internal and is sometimes difficult to isolate, doctors often recommend practising while urinating on the toilet. Try to contract the muscle until the flow of urine is slowed or stopped and then release it. You should perform 5 to 15 contractions, attempting to hold each contraction for 10 seconds, three to five times daily. Once you have mastered these exercises when passing urine, you will be aware of how to do it and be able to do it without passing urine – you will be able to do it anywhere!

Diabetes

I've just been told that I have diabetes. I looked up all I could on the internet and saw that diabetes always causes impotence. Is this true?

Having diabetes does increase your risk of having ED by up to 40%, but that does not mean that you won't be able to lead a completely full and normal sex life. This does not mean that problems do not occur, as diabetes affects both nerves and blood vessels. It is important to keep your blood sugar level well controlled as this will lessen the likelihood of sexual problems. Most people, both male and female, can look forward to a completely normal sex life. If you have any concerns, then talk to your nurse or doctor when you go for your next checkup. Most treatments available to improve ED are suitable for men with diabetes.

I've had diabetes for 17 years and am now 55 years old. I've lost interest in sex. Is it normal for people with diabetes to suddenly find themselves totally uninterested in sexual intercourse?

No more so than for people without diabetes. The feeling you describe tends to be more common in women than men. You should ask yourself questions as to the quality of your relationship with your partner. Talk to your partner about your problems or have some counselling (see Chapter 6). You might find your own solution, or your doctor could suggest various treatments. It is also possible that your loss of interest is due to erection problems.

I have diabetes and have difficulties in keeping my blood glucose levels stable. Does a low blood glucose affect the ability to achieve or maintain an erection and, more importantly, the ability to ejaculate?

No, unless the blood glucose is very low (less than 2 mmol/l), in which case many aspects of nerve function are impaired and this can affect both potency and ejaculation. These return to normal when the blood glucose is back to normal.

Am I likely to become impotent? I have had diabetes for 5 years and feel that my sex life has deteriorated recently.

There is no doubt that many people with diabetes worry about possible future complications, and many men have loss of potency at the top of their worry list. Our advice is to worry more about keeping your diabetes under control and balanced and less about what the future might hold. By ensuring that you have good control of your diabetes, you are doing everything that you possibly can to avoid trouble in the future, and the chances are that you will steer clear of difficulties throughout your life. Your anxiety about being impotent is potentially the real reason that you are having problems.

Some men with diabetes do become impotent because of problems with the blood supply or the nerve supply to the penis. This usually develops slowly and, even if you are younger, we believe it can be prevented by good blood glucose control.

Lately I have had trouble keeping an erection. Has this anything to do with my diabetes? I also had a vasectomy a few years ago.

This is difficult to answer without knowing more about you and your medical history. Certainly it is unlikely that the vasectomy had anything to do with your current problem. Failure to maintain an adequate erection could occasionally be an early symptom of nerve damage from diabetes (diabetic neuropathy). However, it can just be a symptom of overwork, stress or simply growing older. In order to work out if it is due to your diabetes, you need to be assessed by your nurse or doctor. Even if it is to do with diabetes, there are treatments that will work for you.

After sexual intercourse I recently suffered quite a bad hypo, which shook me up and really freaked my girlfriend who didn't know that I had diabetes! Is this likely to happen again and, if so, what can be done to prevent it?

This form of physical activity can, like any other, lower the blood glucose level and lead to hypoglycaemia. When this happens, and it is not at all uncommon, then the usual remedies need to be taken – more food or sugar beforehand or immediately afterwards. You may find it useful to keep some quick-acting carbohydrate close at hand, perhaps on a bedside table.

It is more important to make sure that your blood sugars are not low before you have sex, especially if you have had any alcohol to drink as alcohol reduces blood sugars.

My husband, who is 55 and has Type 1 diabetes, has been impotent for the past 2 years. Please will you explain his condition as I am worried that my teenage son, who also has diabetes, may also discover that he is impotent.

Impotence or the anxiety of becoming impotent worries most men and is certainly not so rare that we can ignore it. It has been claimed that as many as 40% of men with diabetes might at some stage become impotent, to varying degrees. The majority of men who suffer from impotence usually have a medical reason as to why, but men who are anxious, depressed, overworked, tired, stressed, feeling guilty, or who are grieving, can also suffer from impotence, whether they have a medical condition or not. There are good therapies to help your husband. Any man may find that he is temporarily impotent and there is no reason why men with diabetes should not also experience this. Fear of failure can perpetuate the condition.

Stroke

I suffered a stroke affecting the right side of my body 12 months ago at the age of 40 and now suffer from partial impotence. The onset seemed to coincide not with the stroke but with taking anticoagulants and blood pressure tablets, which I have been taking for 3 months. Would these drugs cause impotence?

A severe stroke can sometimes be associated with impotence. A stroke is often due to narrowing of the arteries inside the head. The arteries elsewhere may also be narrowed and, if those supplying blood to the penis are affected, this could contribute to your impotence.

You are quite right about the question of drugs. Some blood pressure lowering drugs may cause impotence and can interfere with ejaculation. Your ED may not be due to your blood pressure tablets but possibly to having high blood pressure itself. This is a common cause for ED. Ask your GP to try you on other drugs. It would be unwise to stop taking your current drugs before you visit your doctor since this would lead to loss of control of your blood pressure. There are also other blood pressure treatments that your doctor can tell you about. Do not be concerned if your doctor does not change your medication as there are now excellent therapies to help ED, regardless of what has caused it.

Anticoagulant tablets are not known to cause impotence.

After having a stroke, I find making love difficult as I just can't move enough. What can you recommend?

This is now a time for experimenting and finding new sexual positions. Try experimenting around your sleeping position to find out new sexual positions. If you sleep on your back, your partner could go on top, or lying on your side might help. For sex to be comfortable, you will need to make sure that you have enough pillows to support you and that the room is warm. If you suffer from spasms or rigidity in your legs, then sitting in an appropriate chair (without arms) would allow your partner to sit on your penis either facing you or with her back to you.

It would be worth contacting SPOD (the association to aid the sexual and personal relationships of people with a disability – see Appendix 1) for further information and advice.

Depression and stress

Overwork or worry is frequently the cause of lack of interest in sex or even of impotence. Excess alcohol can also cause prolonged lack of potency.

I understand that you can have very little physical function and yet have a good sex life. This is just unfair, as I have good physical health and my partner and I have no sex life. The clinic says it is 'sabotage' by my partner. I am so depressed. What is going on?

Sexual function is dependent on numerous factors ranging from perception of sexual stimuli in the brain, through to the swelling of the genitals with blood. Good physical health is hence one very important component of a good sex life, but by no means the only one. As you suggest, couples who are not in the best of physical health can have a very good sex life, whereas other people who are physically 'fit' can have great trouble with it.

The word 'sabotage' is a very emotive one and places the blame of a sexual dysfunction onto one partner. This is very rarely the case. In the vast majority of people, a sexual problem affects two people and both probably contribute to it.

You mention that you are depressed. Depression is a major contributory factor to sexual dysfunction both as a cause and as an effect. Treatment for depression can also cause sexual dysfunction. For instance, treatment with the SSRIs (selective serotonin reuptake inhibitors), such as Prozac, may cause delayed orgasm.

The way forward is very clearly one that involves both you and your partner. You and your partner need to work towards a solution, without attempting to apportion blame. This work can be done by yourselves or you might find more benefit in seeing a trained psychosexual counsellor (see Chapter 6). Your problems can certainly be helped as long as you both want to resolve the issues within your relationship.

Can stress cause ED?

Yes. Depression, stress, anxiety and fear of poor sexual performance are the commonest causes of psychological ED. If you are suffering from stress then this can affect your desire (libido), and in turn affect your erections. If you are taking antidepressants for the stress, there are some types that affect erectile function and you will need to discuss this with your doctor.

Psychosexual counselling or stress management can help to overcome your ED – ask your GP to refer you to a specialist (see Chapter 6).

Kidney disease

I was convinced that my husband had found somebody else, because he was avoiding having sex with me. I didn't realize he couldn't get an erection anymore, because of his kidney failure. Now I can cope with his loss of interest, but I wish he would still have a hug and a kiss.

Many men who are unable to get an erection are afraid of affectionate cuddling, in case the woman expects them to go further and make love. Physical contact is also a reminder that they are unable to make love 'properly', which might make them think they are not a 'real man' anymore. This is a great pity, because everybody needs the reassurance of affectionate physical contact from time to time.

The first thing is to tell your husband how you feel and what you would like him to do – give you a hug and a kiss so that you feel loved and needed.

You might well benefit from some relationship counselling. An organization like Relate may be particularly helpful – you will find the telephone number for your nearest branch in your local telephone directory, or your GP could refer you to a local counsellor. See also Chapter 6 on *Counselling*.

I have been married for 15 years, and love my wife very much. We had a good sex life up until last year when I became ill with kidney failure. I don't seem to get aroused by her anymore, though I find other women attractive and fantasize about sex with other women. Is that normal?

This is a common reaction in men who have a very loving and caring partner. The role of your partner often changes when you are ill. She becomes more of a mother than a lover, which can affect the way you feel about her and act towards her sexually, since you may need to feel dominant and 'masculine' to become aroused. It is far easier to feel like this in a fantasy relationship. If you are able to talk to your wife about this it may be helpful. If you are not making love at present, your wife may also be fantasizing about sex. She may even have started to think you don't love her any more, especially if you have stopped hugging and kissing each other as well. That would be normal too. If you cannot talk together, you could try seeking help from a counsellor to rediscover your sexual relationship (see Chapter 6).

I am a man in my 50s who has lost all interest in sex with my wife over the last 2 years. Now I have just been told I have kidney failure, and the doctor said that people like me often have sexual problems. I am so relieved! I thought there was something wrong with me!

You are quite right – there is nothing wrong with 'you'. You have not lost your masculinity, you are just suffering from an illness that, for physical reasons, can make you lose interest in sex. When your kidney failure has been sorted, you should work on re-establishing your sex life.

My husband, a dialysis patient, has not made love to me for 2 years, and I was getting desperate with frustration. Finally we saw a counsellor, who asked him if he ever had an erection nowadays. He said that, sometimes in the early mornings, he did for a short time, but I was always fast asleep then and he didn't like to bother me. I wish he had told me! A few days later we were able to make love.

It is good that you have managed to overcome your problems of when you make love and have rekindled your sex life. An erection occurs when extra blood enters the penis, and is not allowed to leave. Your husband's kidney failure has probably been making it difficult for him to get an erection. It is often in the early morning that hormone levels (the chemical substances that help with an erection) are highest and drug levels lowest (some drugs, especially certain blood pressure tablets, have side effects that make it difficult to get an erection), and the possibility of lovemaking is most likely. It often helps if couples chat about their problems, as they may find a way to solve the problem. For example, you did not mind at all being woken up early in the morning to make love.

I've always prided myself on . . . you know . . . 'getting it up'. I'm now on dialysis, and I can still get it up but, I can't keep it up. What's going on? My girlfriend will leave me for someone else unless we can sort this out.

Impotence occurs in up to 90% of male dialysis patients. Even though kidney failure causes impotence, there may be other factors involved. For example, both diabetes and a poor blood supply to the penis (which can be linked to renovascular disease) can contribute. The treatment depends on what has caused the problem in your case. Your doctor will want to make sure that you are not underdialysed, so that your general condition improves. If you are anaemic, you should be given erythropoietin (which will increase the number of red blood cells in your blood) and/or iron supplements. Making the anaemia better gives you more energy, and can help with your sexual problems.

It is also a good idea to check all the medicines that you are taking, since some tablets can affect a man's ability to have an erection. If this is the case, an alternative tablet may be found. If you do have low testosterone levels, then you may be started on testosterone replacement therapy – this might improve your desire (libido) but it won't improve your erections, so you will need to seek other forms of treatment. Your renal doctor will be able to advise you on suitable treatments that will help to improve your erections.

Treatments are discussed in Chapters 5 to 10. If this is causing problems within your relationship, then you would benefit from being referred to a counsellor.

If I have a kidney transplant, will my erections return to normal?

Yes, as a general rule sexual function, including the ability to get an erection, improves after a transplant. It is not always the case, because in some men the problem is caused by other factors, such as relationship problems, diabetes, blood pressure or medication that you might be on, which are not cured by transplantation.

I am very tired and worn out after my haemodialysis sessions and don't really feel like lovemaking. My partner feels that I have gone off her and doesn't seem to understand that I do love her, but just don't feel like making love. What can I do?

Patients on dialysis often feel very tired, especially following a session on the machine. Other causes of loss of sex drive can be depression, anaemia or a change in roles between you and your partner. It is important your partner knows she is still valued. Try to show her that you love her. You could also try planning something romantic, like buying a bunch of roses, on the days when you are not tired!

When men don't feel like making love, they sometimes stop all physical contact – no more hugs, kisses or signs of affection. Partners need to feel that they are loved, so talk to yours and let her know how you feel.

Don't give up – there are solutions. Discuss the problem with your doctor or nurses when you visit the clinic next.

Cancer

Last February I was diagnosed with cancer, which was very upsetting and I think caused me to go off sex. Does cancer cause sexual problems?

Finding out that you have been diagnosed with cancer can have both physical and psychological affects on erectile function. Not all cancers will have a physical effect on your erections but you might experience loss of desire (libido), especially if you have to have chemotherapy or radiotherapy.

You are going to experience a lot of anxieties whilst you are coping with the diagnosis and the treatment of cancer. This in turn will have a knock-on effect with your sexual responses. Talk to somebody if you are experiencing any sexual difficulties – your GP will be able to advise you on where you can go for support and information. If you have a partner, it is important to talk together about how you feel.

If you have to have surgery to remove the tumour, for example removal of your prostate, the surgeon will try not to damage the nerves that affect erectile function (this is called a nerve-sparing prostatectomy), but it is not always possible. Don't despair if your cancer treatment has caused problems – there are plenty of options open to you that have worked for others.

Could you explain what this 'nerve-sparing radical prostatectomy is?

Prostate surgery can cause impotence, usually from damage to the nerves or the blood supply that are essential for erections. Over the last decade surgeons have been able to identify the nerves involved in erections and have developed surgical approaches that do not harm these nerves during surgery.

There used to be 100% risk of having ED following a radical prostatectomy. With nerve-sparing surgery this is now down to 30–60%, but is dependent on the age of the patients, the extent of the tumour and the surgical technique. The best thing is to discuss this with your doctor – she or he will be in the best position to advise you on all the options open to you.

4
Relationships

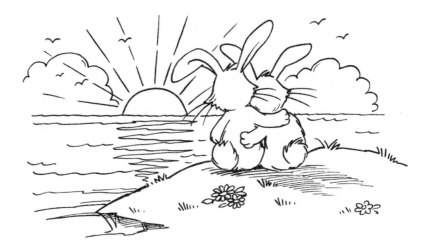

Sexual dysfunction affects both people in a relationship. This is particularly true if there is little communication between partners regarding their problem. For instance, a man may have made love with his partner weekly over the course of their relationship for many years, and then suddenly stop doing so without explaining why. His partner will naturally feel rejected and might consider that his affection has gone elsewhere, causing much hurt and anger. Such a breakdown might even lead to people not touching each other at all in order to avoid potentially stressful sexual circumstances. Equally, if a woman appears to have lost interest in having sex, or the sex appears to be painful for her, this can cause a sexual problem in a man, which may show as a loss of interest in having sex, ED or rapid ejaculation. This is why many couples who suffer sexual dysfunction benefit from relationship therapy, rather than therapy restricted only to sexual practices.

My partner can't get an erection and blames me. How can that possibly be right?

No one is to blame for sexual problems. Equally problems are not 'his' or 'hers' but are problems affecting both people in a sexual relationship. Therefore, rather than labelling a problem his or hers, a sexual partnership needs to work together so that the problem can be sorted.

Sexual problems in one partner can cause sexual problems in the other: 30% of women who have vaginismus (where the vagina closes tightly) have partners who have ED. Similarly, a women who has lost interest in sex may cause her partner to lose interest or develop ED. The key is clearly to communicate with each other about feelings and problems.

My husband has always wanted to make love to me and now he won't even cuddle me. What is the matter?

Having sex is very important to most men and, when it ceases, many feel too embarrassed to talk about the issue, even to their partners. Although people may have been together for 30–40 years and have had regular sex throughout their lives, it is a common story to hear that they have never discussed the issue of sex or sexuality. This lack of communication can lead to a man avoiding the potentially embarrassing situation of not being able to gain an erection rather than discussing his problems, so he avoids having not only sex, but also any form of physical contact with his wife. This often leads his partner to presume that he must be having an affair because, if he doesn't wish to have sex, then he must be having sex with someone else. This presumption can clearly lead to disharmony in an otherwise solid relationship.

I read in a book that men and women work on different cycles of sexual desire, as a rule with women having perhaps two or three high peaks of desire in a month, and men perhaps ten smaller peaks. The snag is that my boyfriend wants sex much more often than I do and I feel that I never get to reach my full potential of sexual desire before we make love, so I feel cheated. What can I do?

Sex is all about good communication and it is vitally important that partners are able to discuss their likes and dislikes, and wishes and disappointments with each other. One suggestion would therefore be that you talk to your partner about your feelings and about this seeming disparity in sexual desire. Interestingly, the authors have looked after many patients where such an imbalance existed. When the issue was finally aired between patients, it resulted in them both saying, 'Oh, I thought we were having sex that often because that's what you wanted', i.e. fulfilling what you suspect to be your partner's wishes, without actually confirming them. The next stage after the discussion would then be to reach a compromise, both on how often you have and the type of sex, so that you both feel that you're being satisfied, and it should then be a mutually fulfilling sexual relationship.

My wife left me because I was impotent and my doctor said that there is nothing he can do for me – why was I not told about any treatments?

We are surprised that your doctor said that there was nothing to offer you because, even for those people who think that they are completely impotent, there are now several treatments that can be tried.

It must be very upsetting to think that your marriage broke up on account of your impotence. In our experience, most wives are sympathetic and understanding about impotence (whatever the cause), provided that both partners can talk about the matter in an open manner. We have known frank discussions lead to an increase of affection within marriage. Keeping things bottled up leads to the aggression and resentment that emerges from your question.

I work long hard hours and my wife has never wanted for anything. My work sometimes stops me from being interested in sex and my partner really lets me know about it. I think it's my problem, not hers. Do you agree?

A sexual problem affects two people. It may make it difficult for your wife to achieve sexual fulfilment and may indeed lead to a sexual problem in her as well; or your sexual problem may actually be due to a sexual problem in your wife. For instance, you might have developed erection problems if intercourse causes pain for her or she is uninterested in having sex with you.

A common situation would be if you have been with your partner for many years, and then developed erection problems because of blood vessel disease. You might feel uncomfortable discussing the issue with her and find it easier to avoid a potentially embarrassing situation by avoiding contact with her completely. For instance, by sitting up later than she does at night you avoid going to bed at the same time, or even avoid touching and cuddling her. If your wife does not understand what is happening, she will very naturally feel rejected and indeed may feel that you must be having an affair, or at the least has lost interest in her. This common scenario emphasizes the importance of communication in a relationship, as it could be said that having good sex is equivalent to good communication between partners.

I am having problems with my girlfriend and feel that she would prefer a more active sex life. If my erections were better, I am sure that my relationship would be better.

Sex is very important in any relationship. Many people blame a deterioration in their relationship on decreased sexual ability and, if this is the case, then clearly treating erection problems can alleviate this cause of problems in a relationship. However, more often, it is a deterioration in the relationship itself generally that leads to a deterioration in sex life. Clearly in this case, giving you a pill to help you with your erections will not lead to an improvement in your relationship. Relationships and the sexual part of them need to be worked at. They need to have time given to them, with the cooperation from both of you. Sexual dysfunction is not something that occurs in one partner, nor affects only one partner. It is something that needs to involve both partners in a relationship, as it affects both of them.

I have been on HRT for a few years and still feel sexy and want to make love to my husband. He is the same age as me (56) but has little desire to have sex now, and when he does, his erections don't last long enough to satisfy me. Is this common?

This is one of the good effects of HRT for women, in that it replaces the hormone oestrogen, which is reduced following the menopause. I expect that your husband feels rather worried about your renewed desire for sex, especially if he is having problems himself. It can cause a vicious circle, where the worrying causes more problems and the problems cause more worrying. Talk to your GP because you can get a referral if necessary. This is likely to be a more common problem as HRT is prescribed regularly for menopausal women. There is a wealth of information about HRT in the bookshops, the internet and, of course, from your doctor. Just talking to your husband about your needs will help – foreplay and other forms of stimulation can be very good and will help to relieve his stress of not 'satisfying' you.

My husband went for years with no desire to have sex with me. Now this is back, but I've got used to having no intercourse. What should I do?

Men and women frequently have different aspirations in a sexual relationship. For a man, frequently, it is getting an erection and having sex with his partner. However, for a woman, it is commonly the closeness and intimacy associated with a sexual relationship, rather than the focus of sex itself. If your periods have now stopped (postmenopausal), you might have a dry vagina because your oestrogen levels will be lower, which can make penetrative sex uncomfortable. This difference in goals highlights the importance of communication in a relationship and, no matter how embarrassing, you should talk about sex with him and what each of you does or does not want to do in a sexual relationship. This then opens up the opportunity of a compromise so you can both be satisfied.

5
Treatments

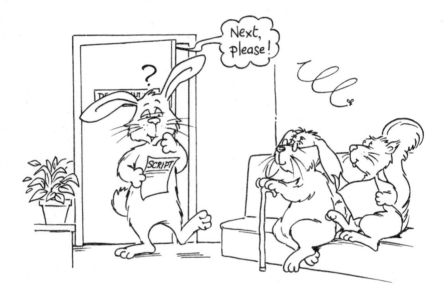

As explained in the section on the causes of impotence, there are various treatments available, each of which will be discussed in separate chapters. The first of these categories is treatment aimed at 'psychological' problems focusing on help with thoughts and beliefs that can affect sexual function. The second group is aimed at 'physical' treatments, including medicines that can be taken by mouth or injected directly into or inserted into the tip of the penis, vacuum pumps and finally surgery. The box opposite shows exactly what is on offer at present. But we begin with some general questions that we are often asked about treatment.

Treatments available for impotence

- Counselling
- Medical oral treatments for erections
  - Viagra
  - Uprima
  - Levitra
  - Cialis
- Medicines directly applied to the penis
  - MUSE
  - Caverject dual chamber/vials
  - Viridal duo
- Surgery – implants
- Vacuum pumps

Will impotence treatments bring back my sexual desire for my partner?

Many men complain to their doctors that they have lost interest in having sex, when indeed the primary problem is that they have ED and avoid sexually arousing situations to avoid embarrassment. If this is happening to you, then effective treatment for ED should bring back some sexual desire. However, if a loss of desire is the primary problem, then there is no evidence that giving any of the licensed therapies for sexual dysfunction will improve your desire. When, for instance, Viagra was first licensed, there was a worry that it would be used as an aphrodisiac by both men and women. While people may have experimented with the drug in this way, the vast majority who use Viagra use it for ED. Lack of 'libido' or desire may be caused by low testosterone levels and your doctor will have assessed these by a blood test should he or she think it necessary.

Are impotence treatments painful?

Pain from treatments varies. A small percentage of people taking Viagra (see Chapter 7 on *Medical oral treatments*) complain of headache and this can happen following apomorphine (Uprima) when taken under the tongue (sublingually). With Viagra, again a small percentage of patients complain of 'acid reflux' (see Chapter 7); however, only a tiny percentage of patients stop taking the medication because of this side effect.

The treatments that are injected in to the penis (see Chapter 8) do cause more pain from the insertion of the needle (although this is only small, as the needle is tiny); however, some people complain of postinjection pain from the acidity of the solution.

Medicated Urethral System for Erection (MUSE) (Chapter 8) can also cause pain when the pellet is inserted; it can also be painful when the drug dissolves in the urethra and sets up a burning sensation.

Do I have to pay for treatment, or can I get it on the NHS?

This depends on whether your problem is one listed in 'Schedule 11' (see below). The government has stated which people can or cannot have an NHS prescription for treatment for ED and this purely depends on the physical reasons for your impotence. Even if you qualify for free prescription, you will still have to pay for your ED treatment if you don't qualify under Schedule 11. If you don't have one of the illnesses or diseases that Schedule 11 recognizes, you should have to pay only for the medication or pumps and not for the GP's consultation time or for a private prescription.

At the time of writing, the illnesses or diseases that are eligible for NHS prescriptions are as follows:

- prostate cancer and prostatectomy
- spinal cord injury
- renal failure
- diabetes
- multiple sclerosis

- single gene neurological disorders
- spina bifida
- polio
- Parkinson's disease
- radical pelvic surgery or pelvic injury.

This may alter in the future so seek advice from your GP, the Sexual Dysfunction Association (formerly the Impotence Association) or local clinic for more up-to-date information. For people with this limited number of diseases and ED, GPs can prescribe treatment, and there is no need for them to prove that the condition is the cause of the ED.

If you do not have one of the above specific diseases, don't feel that you are the only one being excluded. Depending on the particular clinic, as many as 80% of people could be excluded from this list. Most doctors feel that there is no medical justification for this list, and that this is purely a financial decision taken by the government in order to restrict funding, despite ED being a serious medical problem. The regulation does allow for men, who do not have one of the listed conditions but who suffer severe distress from their ED, to receive treatment on the NHS. The assessment of severe distress is made by the GP who considers whether ED has:

- a significant disruption to normal social and occupational activity;
- a marked effect on mood, behaviour, social and environmental awareness;
- a marked effect on interpersonal relationships.

You would be referred to a specialist for confirmation; initial and follow-up treatment has to be prescribed by the specialist, not by the GP. Schedule 11 (the list of conditions) also allows all men who were receiving treatment on and prior to 14 September 1998 to receive all treatments for ED on the NHS at current prescription prices. People who do not fall into any of these categories must get their medication by means of a private prescription, which they will be given at no charge by their GP or their hospital consultant.

How do the costs of the different treatments compare?

At the time of writing, Uprima is priced slightly below Viagra, Levitra and Cialis, with injections and MUSE being significantly more expensive.

I've got this far and I do think that I have ED. How can I get the necessary support?

Your GP or Practice Nurse should be the first port of call. They are highly skilled in a wide variety of medical and social problems and will be able to give you advice, or to refer you to the local experts in this field. If, for whatever reason, you do not feel comfortable discussing your sexual problems with your GP, Appendix 1 gives a list of advice services or websites, such as the Sexual Dysfunction Association (formerly the Impotence Association) helpline, which can give you information about the treatment that you want. Be reassured that you are by no means the only person with sexual dysfunction. It may be very embarrassing for some people to mention this in the first instance. However, the sooner that you bring up the problem with your GP, the sooner treatment can be started and information given that will help you and your partner to resume a satisfactory sex life. Depending on your local services, you might be able to get help from your local sexual health clinic without being previously referred from your local doctor.

I'm at my wits' end and feel so depressed about not being able to satisfy my partner (by the way I'm gay). Our physical relationship means a lot to both of us. If my impotence can't be cured, what should I do then?

Therapies for ED are successful for most of the time. You need to talk to your GP or practice nurse, or be referred appropriately to talk about your options. It doesn't make any difference what your sexual preferences/practices are. It is more important for you and your partner to be happy with your choice of therapy. Therapies are not dependent on sexual practices but are affected by a medical history and other medications being taken.

Most people now choose an oral treatment. If this is unsuccessful, you could then move on to other therapies, either injections or MUSE. If these therapies fail, ask your local doctor to refer you to the specialists who deal with sexual dysfunction in your area. This may be a specialist unit that specifically deals with ED or it may be a health specialist for a particular illness if the ED has been caused by that, such as a cardiologist (for blood pressure or heart attack), diabetologist (for diabetes), or a urological surgeon for prostate problems, pelvic cancer or any other general conditions). The latter also deals with operations to help with erection problems, such as the insertion of a penile prosthesis (see Chapter 10) and will discuss the pros and cons of having such an operation as this with you.

Frankly, I'm 58 and just think it is silly to go through all this at my age. It's so embarrassing and I can't be bothered. Is it normal not to want to be treated?

There is no right or wrong answer to this question, but only what is right for you and your partner. A European survey reported that less than 20% of men would seek help for impotence if they experienced it, but this was before the introduction of Viagra. Many people come forward, not to get treated, but to find out what is happening to them, to exclude major disease and to find out what the treatment options are. With correct guidance and treatment, and a positive approach, a good sexual life can be experienced during your 60s, 70s and even 80s.

6
Counselling

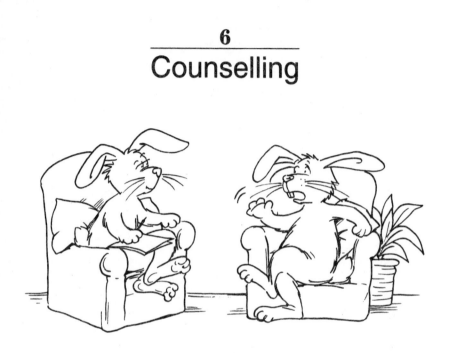

Many men find the idea of psychosexual counselling frightening. However, counselling can vary from simple information giving, through a variety of techniques that will allow a man and his partner, if appropriate, to understand the reasons behind his sexual problem and to develop strategies to deal with these problems.

I'll try anything, even though I'm a bit sceptical about counselling. Where can I find out about it?

Your GP can refer you or your local Sexual Health Clinic will know where you can receive counselling, or they might offer that service themselves. RELATE offer a counselling service for couples with sexual problems (see Appendix 1). You could also look in your local Yellow Pages, as services are not evenly distributed across the country.

I'm on Social Support and am not well off. Can I get counselling on the NHS?

Counselling is available on the NHS, but not in all regions of the country. If it is available locally you will need a referral from your GP, but you may find that there is a waiting list.

To be honest, talking about my failure to have proper sex with my girlfriend is something I can't face. Is it natural that I feel I can't talk to anyone about this?

Yes, this is perfectly normal. The hardest step in dealing with a sexual problem is admitting that there is a problem. Sometimes the best person to talk about it with is your wife or partner, but often men avoid the whole sexual situation by not discussing it, and this makes their partner feel rejected (see next section). Men may also feel reluctant to discuss a sexual problem with their GP. Be reassured that this is a problem that will be taken seriously by your doctor, as it is rated by people as one of the most important things affecting your feelings about life. If you still feel that you cannot mention it to your doctor or practice nurse, information is available from a variety of sources listed in Appendix 1.

My partner has a problem. I know it, and he knows it, but he will not talk about it. Could our GP help?

The most difficult step to take for any man with sexual dysfunction is the first one, and that is acknowledging that he has a problem. He may not wish to acknowledge this fact for several reasons – for instance, feeling that he is a failure, feeling that his partner will no longer love him, feeling that he is the only one that this has ever happened to and is therefore isolated, and feeling that there is no possible answer – but of course there are lots of treatments and he is not alone.

There are several ways that he can get some information about his particular condition:

- He may feel comfortable discussing it with his GP. This has several advantages. The GP will know him very well and may be able to link it with other symptoms, and thus be able to diagnose any sort of underlying problem. The doctor will also be well aware of his social circumstances and therefore of the psychological issues that could have affected his sexual functioning. However, many people do not feel comfortable in raising this issue with their GP. If this is the case, there are other options.
- The Sexual Dysfunction Association (formerly the Impotence Association) – see Appendix 1 – provides a helpline where people can get information; they also have many very valuable leaflets giving basic information about particular conditions, plus some reasonably priced books, written in easy-to-understand language. You have started on the right path by buying the book you are reading now!
- The internet can be useful – we give some sites in the Appendices.

My new partner is much younger than me – I'm 45 and she's only 20. I'm terrified that she will laugh at me or leave me if I try and get help for my ED. Do I have to involve my partner in the treatment? If so, how does this help?

You don't have to involve your partner in the treatment of sexual dysfunction. However, obviously if a problem affects two people, then it would seem more sensible for you to involve her in the treatment, or at least in the discussion of treatment for this issue. Men and women have different expectations of sex and it may be that you are concerned that your problem is really a problem for her, whereas she may have a completely different perspective. One of the cornerstones of psychosexual therapy is getting partners to discuss their sexual problems and letting them find a way forward for themselves. Sex doesn't have to last for any given length of time or be of any given frequency. It needs to be the right thing for you in your particular sexual relationship.

Involving her would have several clear advantages:

- It aids communication about sex in a relationship. Such a lack of communication may indeed be the actual cause of some sexual problems.
- It stresses that a sexual problem is not one that is the fault or problem of just one partner, but is a problem for both partners and needs to 'solved' together.
- Any behavioural exercises such as sensate focus or stop-start (see later question) will be difficult to do without the help and understanding of a partner.
- Anyone can make assumptions about the type and frequency of sex that their partner wants, and communication about sex will clearly help.
- What is perceived by one partner in a sexual relationship as being a problem may not be seen as a problem by the other one.

Even so, if you don't want to involve your partner, you should still seek help.

My husband is a GP and we haven't had sex for 7 years. He is embarrassed to talk to his own GP about this as he has been seeing him for many years and considers him a friend. Can he see a different GP, or another specialist?

Yes, if your husband is in a practice where there are many partners, he could see another doctor regarding this particular problem. If he goes to a single-handed GP, then this is more difficult, but he can access care through other local service providers and the telephone numbers and websites that might be helpful are listed in Appendix 1 of this book. However, you should urge him to consider carefully discussing this issue with his GP, who will know him very well and know his other illnesses and medication, and be the person best placed to advise him. Please reassure your husband that he is by no means the only man that this happens to and, particularly as men get older, ED is a very common problem. He should not be embarrassed about this and instead he should be urged to seek treatment.

When I was rock climbing I fell and damaged my spine. I was in hospital for 6 months and now suffer from both short- and long-term memory loss. I can now walk but the accident has left me with some weakness in my legs. According to my girlfriend, I had no problems obtaining or maintaining erections before the accident but since the accident I haven't had any form of erection. My consultant says it is all in my head but I don't think it is. They are going to refer me to see a counsellor. Do you think I should go?

Yes. Without being able to talk to you and get an in-depth history from you, it is hard to know if your ED is due to psychological reasons (in your head) or organic reasons (climbing accident) and a psychosexual therapist will be able to do just that.

There is probably a physical component to your ED but the therapist or counsellor will be able to refer you if they feel you need a medical consultation. See also the section on *Spinal cord injuries* in Chapter 2.

Psychosexual treatment

The words 'psychosexual counselling' seem rather daunting to many people, but really it is only treatment via a counsellor who will talk you through your problems and suggest ways that they might be overcome. As in all treatments there are advantages and disadvantages, some of which are listed in the box opposite.

My doctor told me first to have some 'psychosexual therapy' when I discussed my ED with him. What is this?

The majority of men with ED have a combination of physical and psychological components causing their sexual problems. Hence,

---

Advantages and disadvantages of psychosexual therapy

Advantages

- No drugs are needed.
- Both partners will be able to understand their problems better.
- Partners will communicate better following therapy.
- Time can allow things to naturally get back to normal.

Disadvantages

- Treatment is not always available on NHS.
- Treatment can be time-consuming – there is no 'instant' recovery.
- During consultations, subjects may be raised that you would prefer not to discuss.
- If you attend alone, without your partner, treatment is not usually so successful.

---

most men could benefit from psychosexual counselling either in addition to drugs or as therapy on its own. However, psycho-sexual counselling does not work for everybody. It is not available in many parts of Britain on the NHS and thus cost can be a factor. It is slow, it is time-consuming and it needs effort put in from you, as the counsellor will not be fixing the actual problems for you, but attempting to lead you along a path that will enable you to come to a satisfactory conclusion for yourself.

A lot of people are scared by the thought of psychosexual counselling. However, like many things in life, this term covers a broad spectrum. It might be as simple as giving out information: for instance, many men state at some stage during their consultation that indeed the real problem they have sexually is that their penises are far too small. In reality, 99% of men have a penis that is more than adequate for sexual intercourse. Another commonly held fallacy is that men should want to make love all the time. The real answer is that over 50 years of age, men in

Britain make love on average once to twice per week. Some sexual therapy can also involve graduated exercises, such as sensate focus or behavioural therapy to stop rapid ejaculation (see next question). This involves a counsellor taking you and your partner, if appropriate, through a graduated series of exercises, which will enable you to control your erection and ejaculation. It is only in the minority of cases of people who have a sexual dysfunction that many sessions of psychotherapy are necessary.

Sensate focus treatment

My counsellor has recommended sensate focus therapy for us, as my husband has problems with erections. He is violently against it but I'm quite happy to try anything that will stop him getting depressed and drinking as much as he does. What will this involve?

Sensate focus is a structured programme of exercises, originally described by Masters and Johnson in the 1960s. The aim is to learn to feel and respond pleasurably to simple touching and stroking, and to communicate what sensory experiences are pleasurable. From stroking and touching each other's bodies in areas away from the genitals, couples progress to touching each other's genitals and finally to penetration in a controlled position.

In *stage 1*, the non-genital stage, the man and the woman in turn are encouraged to caress, fondle each other all over the body but not in the genital area. It is a vital part of this stage that the partners tell each other where and how they want to be touched. When the couple feel comfortable with this exercise, they are then encouraged to move to *stage 2*, where the genital area becomes the focus of the attention. It is important to realise that the pattern of sexual likes and dislikes are infinitely variable from man to man and woman to woman, and you must both talk to and listen to each other. The aim of this stage is to become competent at pleasuring your partner in a way that excites both of you. Your husband will probably get an erection during this stage. This stage can be continued for some weeks.

In the final *stage 3*, the controlled intercourse exercise, you will be advised to kneel astride your partner, facing him. In this position, you can control the depth, direction and speed of penetration, allowing your partner to concentrate on his own sensations. At first you may be advised not to move at all, then slowly to increase the sensations by increasing the motion of your vagina on his penis.

After this controlled stage of intercourse (also know as the 'penile' or 'vaginal containment' stage), you can gradually increase the activity in order to gain the maximal stimulation for both you and your partner. If his problems recur during these exercises, retrace your steps to a stage where you both feel confident and begin the process again.

Cognitive treatment

I am going to a counsellor soon to talk about a cognitive approach to treatment. How is this different to the sensate focus therapy you mentioned above?

Some counsellors suggest this especially if you have talked about negative thoughts and actions when you are trying to make love. Anxiety and fear will interfere with sexual function. Sensate focus therapy is known as 'behavioural therapy' in that the process is trying to change your behaviour and the way you approach your lovemaking. 'Cognitive therapy' on the other hand relates to your thought processes and will help you to confront your fears and negative thoughts and eventually overcome them.

7
Medical oral treatments

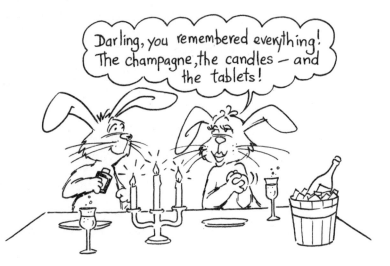

Treatment for ED has been revolutionized since the introduction of Viagra. Prior to this, men were limited to treatments pushed into their penises. While these treatments are effective for many, the majority of men would prefer to take something by mouth to help with their erections. There are now four licensed oral treatments for ED in the UK – sildenafil (Viagra), apomorphine (Uprima), vardenafil (Levitra) and tadalafil (Cialis). These treatments, as well as other drugs that have been used to treat ED, will be discussed in this chapter. First, we discuss where hormonal treatment fits in.

Hormonal treatment

The consultant at the hospital suggested I 'think about' testosterone. Will taking testosterone replacement therapy help my impotence?

Testosterone is the hormone responsible in the main part for sexual drive and the development of what are called 'secondary' male sexual characteristics (see next question). Erections are dependent on getting blood into the penis and therefore dependent on healthy blood vessels and nervous system sending the messages that open up the blood vessels. Erections themselves are **not** dependent on testosterone. See Chapter 2 for the role that hormones play. The idea is that testosterone replacement therapy may well help to increase sexual drive, but there is no evidence that it improves erections. Against the possible benefits of testosterone replacement, you will have to balance the potential danger of aiding the development of hormone-dependent cancers, such as prostate cancer.

I was told by my GP that my testosterone is abnormally low, but that came as a surprise to me (I'm 59). How would I know if my testosterone level is low?

Very rarely, young men do not develop any secondary sexual characteristics such as voice deepening, appearance of bodily or pubic hair, muscle bulk and adult genitals, and will also have decreased sexual drive, and these may all be signs of an abnormally low testosterone level. If you are an adult man with normal secondary sexual characteristics, the most likely reasons you might have for a blood test for testosterone levels being low are:

- that the test has been taken in the wrong part of the day, as the testosterone level varies significantly from morning to night;
- that the protein binding testosterone in your blood is high

because you are overweight or have consumed more than average amounts of alcohol;

- because you are an older man – testosterone levels fall with age. This decrease in levels with age has led some researchers to describe this period as the 'andropause', the male equivalent of the female menopause.

You mention the 'andropause' – I was reading about this the other day and I certainly feel changes in my mood at the moment. Do you think that men go through something similar to the menopause then?

Doctors have found these decreased testosterone levels in older men. The symptoms of the andropause are, however, far more variable, and happen over a far longer time scale. Although they are vague and poorly defined, they can include nervousness, depression, inability to concentrate, fatigue, insomnia, reduced desire for sex (libido) and hot flushes. So the possible benefits of testosterone replacement therapy are not nearly as clear cut as they are for HRT in women.

What is testosterone replacement therapy, and are there any side effects to this treatment?

Androgens are a group of hormones present in both men and women, the most well known of which is testosterone. However, although a few doctors do prescribe it for the treatment of ED, there is no really good evidence that it works.

The side effects of androgen replacement therapy are a deepening of the voice and increased facial hair, as well as an increase in muscle bulk. These are clearly problems more worrying to women than to men. However, in men there is at least one very dangerous possible side effect: androgen replacement therapy can increase the likelihood of men developing prostate cancer and, if it is to be given, then prostate-specific androgen blood tests must be made regularly so that your doctor can keep an eye on the risk of you developing prostate cancer.

Do discuss with your doctor or at the ED clinic the possible benefits and risks of testosterone replacement therapy. For some men results have been very helpful, but the choice will ultimately be up to you.

Sildenafil (Viagra)

Viagra was a major breakthrough for patients and doctors living with and managing erectile dysfunction, but it does not suit or help everyone with erection problems. When there is sexual stimulation, be that by touch, or sight, or smell, or whatever turns a man on, this is perceived by a certain area in the brain and then a cascade of chemical 'messengers' is sent out, which leads to the blood vessels supplying the penis opening up. One of these messengers is called 'cyclic GMP', and it is broken down by an enzyme called 'phosphodiesterase'. The medications such as Viagra, Levitra or Cialis work by blocking this phosphodiesterase and thus leading to an increased period where the blood vessels will be dilated. The way the drug works is very important for men regarding how it is used. It is only effective when there is sexual stimulation! The drug will not be successful if there is no stimulation, i.e. a man takes the medication and then awaits an erection before attempting any sort of sexual contact. Many men claim that Viagra has failed for them because they have either taken it at too lower a dose, or not often enough, or they have taken it without any sexual stimulation.

At present Viagra is taken orally (by mouth) and, because of the relatively slow digestive process, it may be an hour or two before the drug produces its effects – certainly an issue in planning for sex. It affects not just the penis, but potentially could affect other parts of the body. As with most drugs, not everyone will benefit, although Viagra has been found to produce firmer, more frequent and longer lasting erections in the majority of men who have taken it. Doses are 25, 50 and 100 mg, taken 1 hour before sexual foreplay, and its effect lasts for 2–3 hours.

Advantages and disadvantages of Viagra

Advantages

- Having satisfying sex should not be denied to older men. Viagra has been shown to help problems with ED in this group. Mild to moderate side effects seem to be similar in older and younger age groups, and your GP will be able to discuss these with you.

- Ability to penetrate partners is significantly increased from a few times to most times for patients receiving 100 mg Viagra.

- Ability to maintain an erection after you have penetrated your partner should significantly increase.

- Viagra restores erections to a level almost that of men without ED, but it doesn't have any effect on sexual desire. So, although Viagra will help you to gain an erection with sexual stimulation, it may not have any effect on sexual desire (libido) if other things, such as relationship problems, are affecting that desire.

- Studies have shown that about 85% of attempts at sexual intercourse are successful following Viagra.

- The effect of Viagra does not appear to wear off the more you use it.

- Viagra can significantly improve the erectile response in patients with ED of no known physical cause. One study showed improvement in nearly 90% of men.

- When men's partners were questioned on partner satisfaction, it seems that Viagra significantly improves satisfaction with their sex life.

- Viagra has been on the market for some years now. So far it has shown a good safety record. Only 1% of men have discontinued taking Viagra because of side effects (see the section on side effects below).

- If you are trying for a baby, there has been no suggestion in any of the extensive studies on Viagra that it does any harm either to a man's partner, or to a resultant pregnancy, or to the baby.

Advantages and disadvantages of Viagra (continued)

Disadvantages

- It must not be taken by people taking nitrates.
- If you have had liver failure, eye disorders and certain other illnesses, you must discuss the suitability of Viagra for you.
- Its effects are slower than the injected type of drugs.

Oral therapy is now prescribed in over 90% people with ED, and studies are showing that 70% of these achieve satisfaction. In one study of couples, where 87% of the men rated Viagra as 'somewhat satisfactory to very satisfactory', nearly 30% of their partners considered the treatment 'unsatisfactory', mostly because of their own lack of sexual interest.

We get many questions about this drug. Some of its attributes are listed in the box.

All the junk email I get on my email account tell me that I can buy stuff from the USA that will work straight away. Is there an immediate-acting tablet?

At present, no there is not. Tablets that are taken under the tongue, or potentially in the future by nasal spray, will get into the bloodstream and act faster than tablets that are taken by mouth and swallowed, which need to be absorbed into your bloodstream to work.

All of the tablets that are presently licensed and indeed will be licensed in the near future require you to be sexually stimulated to work. The gap phase between taking a tablet and an erection developing would therefore be valuable for you and your partner to engage in the sort of foreplay that makes you both ready to enjoy making love.

Viagra sounds the perfect solution to my problems, which have affected my relationship with my new partner. How often can I use Viagra?

The recommended frequency of taking tablets is not more than once every 24 hours. There is no restriction on how many times a week you could use Viagra, but if you are getting it on the NHS, most GPs will limit their prescribing to one tablet per week as this is the recommendation in Schedule 11. You might find that, after using Viagra successfully to help you get an erection, your erections can also be better the following day. This could be a direct effect of the drug, but could also be due to the tissues in your penis being enlivened by getting a good supply of oxygenated blood in them.

I like to go out to dinner with my wife on Friday nights and have a Chinese meal. Can I take Viagra after a large meal? Would this be safe or sensible?

Taking Viagra after a large meal will slow the absorption of Viagra. What this means is that you may find that the Viagra does not work at all for you, or that it works much slower than it would have done had you taken it on an empty stomach, or after a light meal. In other words, it is safe in that it will have no harmful effects, but it is not sensible!

I am keen to get my love life as good as it was before we had kids, but do not want to go mad, as I have a demanding job. What dose of Viagra will I need?

The effect of Viagra does seem to improve the higher the dosage taken. The maximum dose is 100 mg. You might find that the dose of Viagra you need is dependent on other factors present at the time of intercourse, such as tiredness and stress. If you are unhappy with the first dose you are prescribed, visit your doctor again to discuss whether you could try a higher one.

I have seen the effect of Viagra on my husband, but do not feel stimulated myself. Could I try one of his Viagra tablets. Could women benefit from Viagra as well?

During foreplay and intercourse there are some very similar processes happening in women to those in men, so in theory Viagra could help to enhance sexual response, but so far there have been few studies of women while taking the drug. Women might feel that this shows a very particular gender bias in the testing of such drugs, but at the moment it is not licensed for women!

Viagra appears to improve the blood supply to the whole genital area. With sexual stimulation, this will lead to blood flowing into your clitoris and vulva and potentially make your vagina more slippery (better lubricated). This allows some women to enjoy sexual activity more; however, the majority of women with desire or libido problems don't appear to be helped. Further research in this area is going on and new results become available all the time. If you are interested in the treatment of Viagra in women, discuss this with your doctor or nurse.

There have been other reports of successful pregnancies in women taking Viagra, who were previously unable to have babies. Viagra may cause the lining of the womb to thicken from better nourishment from the bloodstream.

I am not well off, but should like to try Viagra to see if it will help our relationship. Will I have to pay for a private prescription?

Yes, if you don't conform to Schedule 11. A private prescription means that you will have to pay for the cost of the drug, plus whatever sort of percentage increase the pharmacy will put on the medication. Prices charged by retail pharmacies can vary greatly and it would be worthwhile asking your doctor if they know where the cheapest pharmacy is, or ringing round yourself, including the big retail chains. The prescription from the doctor won't cost you anything – the cost for the chemist lies in getting the drug privately rather than on the NHS.

I have a spinal cord injury and I am experiencing difficulty in achieving and maintaining an erection because of the effects of my injury. Will Viagra help improve my erections?

Viagra has been reported as being well tolerated and is effective in 45–60% of men suffering from spinal cord injury (SCI). As long as you are **not** taking any nitrates, there is no reason why you cannot take Viagra, but discuss treatment options with your GP. The side effects of taking Viagra are the same as for men who don't have a SCI (see section below). You may find that the results from Viagra are not as good as other treatments, such as injection therapy, for improving your erections, but this will dependant on your SCI.

Since having a spinal cord injury, I have had poor erections and Viagra didn't help improve them. Are there any other medications that will help?

Don't despair – there are other drugs available to treat ED such as Cialis, Levitra, Uprima (discussed in the following sections), MUSE, injections and vacuum therapy devices (discussed in Chapters 8 and 9). There is more about spinal cord injury in Chapter 2.

I had a car accident, which damaged my back and I'm now in a wheelchair. Could Viagra help me?

Yes. There have been a few studies of Viagra in people with nerve damage. In people with spinal cord injury, the majority had improved erections and preferred Viagra to 'placebo' (where there was no active-ingredient tablet taken). In a study of people with MS, Viagra improved the erection and side effects were mild to moderate. They felt that sex life was considerably better. So, yes, in your case, you should try consulting your GP, who may well prescribe it for you, and see if it improves your sex life.

I am 25 and have MS. I've read in the MS magazine about Viagra for men's impotence recently. Could that help me sexually?

There has been an enormous amount of publicity about Viagra in recent months, and the ways in which it may transform men's sex lives. Fortunately for many men with erection problems, caused by nervous system damage in MS, it may indeed offer some help. (There is more about sexual problems in MS in Chapter 3).

Essentially Viagra acts on blood supply problems in MS and other similar conditions, by helping the penis to fill with blood. Even where nervous system damage is substantial and where erections are very difficult to obtain and sustain, Viagra might be able to help. As many men with MS are younger than those in which side effects with Viagra have happened, there should be fewer problems amongst your age group.

Note that, because of the cost of the drug, and the anticipated large demand for it, the Department of Health has been extremely circumspect about those for whom it can be prescribed via the NHS (see question in Chapter 5 on Schedule 11). However, MS is now one of the designated medical conditions – but there may still be local variations in supply, in addition to clinical reasons for its non-prescription.

Always get advice from your doctor and **do not** buy it on the internet. Viagra is a very safe and effective treatment, provided that you are guided medically – do not experiment without a medical opinion.

I had heart by-pass surgery 18 months ago. Can I take Viagra?

If this operation was successful and you now have no chest pain, then there is no reason for you not to be having sex, or be treated for any sexual dysfunction. If, however, you are still having chest pain, particularly at rest, then this needs to be sorted out before you embark on any physical activity, including having sex. If you are taking nitrates, you must not take Viagra.

Can I take Viagra? I had a stroke a year ago and worry that I might have another, which is not good for my self-confidence with my girlfriend.

The answer to this question is yes, in the vast majority of cases. Strokes can be either due to bleeding into the brain or to the brain not getting enough blood flow because of a blockage in the arteries. Viagra will open up the arteries flowing to the brain, and this results in some men getting a mild headache and a feeling of fullness in the head, following a Viagra tablet. You will need to discuss the safety issue with your GP, but there is no reason why you should not try having sex again after having had a stroke.

I am on tablets for my depression. Could Viagra actually help my depression as well as my sex life?

Depression and sexual dysfunction can be very much a 'chicken and egg' situation because some ED problems could actually cause anxiety and depression, but, in long-standing depression, Viagra is successful in helping people have intercourse. We have discussed psychological problems in Chapter 2.

There is increasing evidence that men who are on anti-depressive treatment, when treated with Viagra, can, in some cases, decrease the amount of antidepressant therapy that they are taking.

If you are on medication called SSRIs (selective serotonin reuptake inhibitors), you should get better erections with Viagra.

I have had diabetes for the past 15 years (I'm 39) and find it very difficult to make love to my wife nowadays because I can't sustain an erection. Would Viagra help me?

It could well do. In one study, Viagra helped over 50% of men with diabetes and ED. The effects did not seem to be affected by age, or how long they had had ED or diabetes. Although the response to Viagra was somewhat less than that seen in other groups, people with diabetes do often have many other problems, such as vascular disease or diabetic neuropathy.

The majority of side effects (see next section) seen with Viagra (e.g. headache, feeling of acidity, congestion in your nose) are not severe and don't last long, so these should not prevent you from trying Viagra.

I have had a kidney transplant and am on medication. Can I take Viagra?

Yes you can. There is no reason why the drugs normally taken after a transplant operation will interact with Viagra. (The only drug that you cannot take with Viagra is the class of drugs called nitrates, which are given to people for their heart pain.)

I had cancer some months ago, which left me rather incapacitated – I now have trouble having sex with my partner. Would Viagra help me?

You do not say what your disability is, but there are various choices open to you. Tablets would still be your first choice: Viagra, Levitra or Cialis, or Uprima (see the following main sections), depending on what medication you are currently taking. However, you could also try other treatments such as injections, MUSE or a vacuum device (see Chapters 8 and 9), if drugs like Viagra do not work for you.

I've had an operation on my prostate and other treatment for cancer. My doctor was very negative about me having Viagra. Was he right to be so?

We know that men who have undergone surgery or radiotherapy for prostate cancer have taken Viagra successfully. Although the best response was seen in men with less severe ED, over half with complete ED were pleased with the effect Viagra had. So you doctor may well be over-pessimistic about it.

Side effects of Viagra

I have been prescribed Viagra but I am nervous about taking it as I don't like pills. What are the side effects?

When Viagra was first released there were several sensationalist newspaper headlines about men dying after taking the medication. These headlines have given many people the impression that Viagra is potentially a dangerous medication. **This is not true.** As men get older their blood vessels narrow and become hardened and inflexible (atherosclerotic). This is the reason that older men (and women) suffer from cardiovascular disease, which leads to, amongst other problems, heart attacks and strokes. It is the same disease process that stops the blood flowing into the penis, and it is therefore logical that people who are having problems with their erections because of this decreased blood flow might also have decreased blood flow to both their hearts and their brains.

In very extensive studies, both before and after Viagra had been launched ('licensed'), there was no suggestion of Viagra causing death. The one exception to this statement is that simultaneous taking of nitrates, which are drugs taken to stop angina (heart pain), or taken close to the time when Viagra is taken, can be extremely dangerous. This is because the Viagra and the nitrates work in the same way, i.e. by opening up the blood vessels. If taken together, the blood vessels can open too much causing the blood pressure to fall dangerously – in some cases this has led to serious problems, including death. However, if we exclude those people who have taken this combination of drugs, there is no sign of any increase in serious problems in people taking Viagra. Indeed, studies in Britain suggest that there may be fewer serious cardiovascular problems in people taking Viagra, compared with those men who are not taking the medication.

The danger therefore for men taking Viagra, as long they are not taking nitrates as well, is not to do with the drug itself, but with the level of energy expended in sexual activity. This level of energy expenditure is about the same as doing light housework, or walking 1 mile in 20 minutes on the level. We are talking here

---

How to reduce the side effects of Viagra

Headaches. Take headache tablets when you take Viagra.

Indigestion or heartburn. Don't take Viagra within 2 hours of eating. Use antacids or try drinking milk. When having intercourse, don't lie on your back.

Visual colour distortion. This can be alarming but is short lived as are all the side effects of Viagra.

---

of sexual activity with a long-standing partner. Sexual activity with a new partner carries with it a greater degree of anxiety and, therefore, a greater energy expenditure – it can be compared to heavy housework such as scrubbing floors, or digging the garden.

Since my doctor put me on Viagra, I've noticed some improvement but I've also had some blinding headaches. Are there other treatments available?

The majority of men who complain of headaches say that these are mild and that they did not take anything for them. Also, the more they use Viagra, the less the headaches become.

If the headaches are severe, try taking an analgesic before taking your Viagra. You can also try Levitra or Cialis. Although the drugs are similar to Viagra, for a reason we don't understand yet some men get fewer headaches than when taking Viagra.

I am taking tablets to lower my blood pressure. Will the Viagra still work for me?

Treatment for high blood pressure does not interfere with Viagra's effects: erections improved in 70% of men on such treatment compared with only 21% of those who received a placebo. If you were taking more than one drug for your high blood pressure, there shouldn't be any more adverse effects than in someone who is not taking any drugs for high blood pressure at all. Some of these blood pressure drugs actually make having an erection difficult (such as beta blockers), so it would be best to eliminate this possibility first, then discuss with your doctor about taking Viagra.

My older brother (I'm 59) had a heart attack recently and I'm worried that, if I take Viagra, I could be in danger too – at the moment I take water tablets for my high blood pressure.

Men who are having treatment for heart conditions, such as nitrates, run the risk of a dangerous further drop in blood pressure if they take Viagra. Older men, perhaps with an underlying undiagnosed cardiac problem, who may not have undertaken any exercise for several years, could find themselves in difficulty with vigorous sexual activity, so it is important that you discuss things fully with your doctor.

People with heart problems, including coronary heart disease, may benefit from Viagra because heart disease, rather than the drugs used to treat it, is the most common cause of ED.

Viagra does not cause heart attacks (nor do penile injections – see Chapter 8), any more than might occur by chance. Before trying it, have a check-up at the doctor's.

My doctor has given me a small pill to put under my tongue if I get breathless and my chest starts to hurt. I'd like to try Viagra. Is there a problem taking both tablets?

Yes, Viagra reacts with nitrates. You have been given nitrates and you **must not** take Viagra at the same time. There are alternative forms of therapy for ED, such as the new oral tablet Uprima (see section below), injections into the penis, or MUSE (see Chapter 8).

Alternatively, you can talk to your doctor about changing to different treatments. Nitrates are for relatively weak angina (chest pain), and have no proven benefit in preventing heart attacks or sudden death. They are used only to help relieve pain and breathlessness. Heart specialists estimate that up to 90% of patients using nitrate therapy could be treated with other drugs, for example felodipine or amlodipine. Once the change has proved successful (2 weeks should be enough time), you can then try Viagra.

The American Heart Association suggests that it is unsafe to take a nitrate within 24 hours of a Viagra dose. You will be advised, if you are taking Viagra, that you should not keep nitrates in the house, to avoid accidentally taking both of these drugs together. If you do take Viagra and have sex, and then experience chest pain, you should stop the sexual activity and either sit or stand while the symptoms ease. If your chest pain does not ease with this rest, then get medical help immediately.

I am 74 years old and still very active. For the last 5 years I have been prescribed various medications for high blood pressure and cholesterol levels, and also for the mild angina from which I occasionally suffer: simvastatin (Zocor) or atorvastatin (Lipitor) for cholesterol, nicorandil (Ikorel) for angina, felodipine (Plendil) and perindopril (Coversyl) for blood pressure, plus baby aspirins. At the same time as starting these drugs I have suffered from ED, although a number of doctors have said that the treatment I am receiving should not have that effect. When I ask if I can take Viagra, I am told by more than one member of the cardiac department in our local hospital that they do not recommend it for anyone with a heart condition such as mine, the reason being, apparently, that they believe Viagra can constrict the blood vessels to the heart and bring on a heart attack. I appreciate that Viagra should not be taken as well as a nitrate medication and would naturally avoid this, but I have never read that it should be banned to everyone with a common heart condition. It would seem to be just a policy decision by our local cardiologist. What do you think?

If you are not on nitrates, and are a fit active man, then there is no reason why you can't take Viagra. There is an oral therapy, Uprima (see next section), which is suitable for men who are taking nitrates. It is similar in one respect to Viagra, i.e. it needs sexual stimulation to work. It is a tablet that is placed underneath the tongue to dissolve and then takes about 20 minutes to work.

As with all treatments it is not a 100% success, but there are other treatment choices. Talk to your doctor about other forms of treatment for ED. Vacuum therapy devices, injections and MUSE are all suitable alternatives for you (see Chapters 8 and 9).

A friend of mine had a heart attack after taking Viagra – it seems dangerous to me. Are the media reports wrong?

There is no increased risk of a heart attack from Viagra – in fact there were fewer cases of heart attack when Viagra was compared with a placebo (this is where people are given a tablet with no active ingredients in it, but they feel that it has had an effect – a 'placebo effect'). Newspapers like headlines. The many millions of people who have taken Viagra safely seem to disprove this unfounded fear.

I'm really terrified of these chest pains that I sometimes get. It really puts me off taking Viagra.

Do not use a nitrate tablet or spray at the same time as Viagra. Stop your activity and sit or stand up. The pain should gradually settle. A glass of whisky or brandy might be helpful. Do not try to have sex again again until you have discussed what happened with your doctor. There are other options available to you that your GP can tell you about.

I am in my late 60s and had a mild heart attack about 7 years ago. My doctor prescribed atenolol and atorvastatin (Lipitor). I started to have ED about 2 years ago. The doctor changed my tablets from atenolol to what he called an ACE inhibitor but I am still having problems. Injections have not helped. I gather Viagra should not be used. Are there alternatives?

This is a very interesting question which raises several important issues. As has been stressed repeatedly in this book, erections are all about getting blood in to the penis. In this case, the same disease process that has blocked the arteries supplying your heart and caused your heart attack has blocked the arteries supplying the blood to the penis. Many people associate their treatment for high blood pressure with ED. The GP in this case was quite correct in changing the medication, as the older drugs, such as thiazide diuretics and beta blockers, are associated with a higher incidence of ED than the newer ones, such as ACE inhibitors and calcium channel blockers. Also, the only reason not to take Viagra is if you are taking nitrates, either in long-acting form or in the form of tablets that go under your tongue to relieve angina. This is because nitrates plus the Viagra (or the newer drugs, Levitra and Cialis, which are similar to Viagra – see the next section), if taken together, can cause your blood pressure to drop very significantly and hence be very dangerous. In your case, you are taking a lipid-lowering agent and an ACE inhibitor, so there is no reason why Viagra should not be used.

If Viagra is not successful, taking apomorphine under the tongue can be tried (see next section).

Although you say that the injections have not worked, it would be worthwhile reconsidering how the injections were used and what dose was given, as most people will respond to injection therapy if the correct dose is administered correctly.

Would taking Valium before using Viagra interfere with Viagra's effects?

The effect of Valium is to calm the nervous system in the body and to make people feel less apprehensive. There is no reason that taking Valium should stop Viagra working. However, regarding your sexual performance, Valium and other drugs used to decrease anxiety can slow down the time taken to ejaculate. Indeed these drugs are used to treat people who have rapid ejaculation. So if you take a normal time to ejaculate and are taking these drugs, you may find that you are slower to ejaculate, or even find it impossible to ejaculate. This does not happen in most men and, if it does happen to you, then you need to discuss it with your GP – do not stop taking your Valium without discussing the problem first.

Vardenafil (Levitra) and tadalafil (Cialis)

The success of Viagra has interested many pharmaceutical companies and there are now two new drugs, which are the same type of therapy as Viagra. They are called vardenafil (Levitra), marketed by Bayer and GlaxoSmithKline; and tadalafil (Cialis), developed by a technology company called ICOS and marketed on a worldwide basis by Eli Lilly.

Levitra and Cialis have the same advantages and disadvantages as Viagra, discussed previously, so the rest of this chapter will try to explain some of the differences between the three therapies.

Now there are other treatments like Viagra on the market perhaps I should try one of the others? Which one should I start on?

As you would expect with second-generation drugs, they do have advantages over Viagra. However, Viagra works and has no significant side effects for most men. Therefore, you will only find out which treatment is best for you by trying them and seeing which one works best.

Each of the three treatments has its own strengths and weaknesses and your doctor or nurse will be able to discuss these with you. The balance will be an individual one between the potential advantages of the newer medications (Cialis and Levitra) compared with the great clinical experience that doctors now have with Viagra.

Do Cialis and Levitra work in the same way as Viagra?

Yes. Cialis and Levitra act in the same way as Viagra by blocking an enzyme called phosphodiesterase-5 (PDE5). This helps the smooth muscles in the penis relax and widen, allowing more blood to enter. Also similar to Viagra, there needs to be sexual stimulation for the drug to be effective. They are 'facilitators' of sexual activity not 'initiators', i.e. they are not aphrodisiacs.

Is any one of these drugs better than the others?

Some effort has been made by reviewers and by pharmaceutical companies to compare data from different clinical trials (with different patient populations) and conclude that Drug A is superior to Drug B for a given population. Such a conclusion must be treated with some reservation until direct comparative studies are done.

At present all that can be said conclusively is that Viagra, Cialis and Levitra are all very effective and very safe drugs for men with ED.

I have been taking Viagra for some time now. Should I change from Viagra to one of the new tablets?

The answer to this question is one that will be different for each man individually. For some, if Viagra has been successful and they are having no serious side effects, they will see no reason to change their medication. However, for others, there will be the urge to experiment and to try the newer compounds to see if they are better.

Do you think the effects of Viagra could be enhanced by taking Cialis or Levitra in combination?

There have been no clinical trials so far looking at the safety or the effectiveness of such combinations, and therefore it cannot be recommended that you try these drugs in combination at this stage. Take your doctor's advice – don't experiment with medicines!

I know that Viagra has been used by some women. Would Levitra or Cialis help female sexual problems?

It is very likely that these drugs will help some women with sexual problems, as Viagra has done. However, at this stage there have been no research trials reported of women taking these drugs, so as yet we cannot recommend that they are taken until there is some scientific evidence of their usefulness in this area.

Levitra

I made an appointment with my doctor to see if I can take Viagra. My doctor has talked to me about Levitra. He said he was going to start me on a 10 mg dosage. Are there others?

Levitra comes in three doses, but your doctor will probably start you on a dose of 10 mg. Some men find they need a higher dose of 20 mg. A lower dose of 5 mg is also available and is the starting dose for men who are over 65.

How do I take Levitra?

Levitra is an oral tablet, which should be swallowed before you start sexual activity. It does not work immediately and should be taken between 30 and 60 minutes before you want to have sex.

The action of Levitra is not normally affected by food (unless you take it with a very fatty meal) nor by alcohol, so you can eat and drink as normal before taking Levitra.

For most men, the first tablet of Levitra is effective in helping produce and maintain an erection, but don't worry if it doesn't work the first time – some men may not have had sex for some considerable time and may feel apprehensive when they try. It is worth taking Levitra again the next time that you want to have sex: some men find that Levitra works better after a few attempts. Once Levitra starts to work for you then it should continue working reliably.

How long does Levitra last?

Most people will probably be able to get an erection 3 or 4 hours after taking Levitra, although it will work best within the first hour.

Levitra helps maintain erections in the majority of men long enough for completion of sexual intercourse. Once intercourse has been finished, the erection will subside as it would do normally. If the erection does not subside within a couple of hours then you should contact your doctor.

If you want to have sex the following day, another tablet of Levitra will be needed. It is recommended that only one dose of Levitra is taken in a 24-hour period.

How safe is Levitra?

All the clinical trials that have been conducted with Levitra show it to be a well tolerated drug. In trials lasting up to a year, no long term side effects have been seen. Some men can experience certain side effects and these are described below.

There are some patients for whom Levitra will not be suitable, in particular anyone who has coronary heart disease and is being treated with nitrates. This includes nitrates that are taken daily to help prevent angina or short-acting nitrates (under the tongue sprays or tablets). Like Viagra, Levitra should never be taken in conjunction with a nitrate. If you are unsure whether you are taking a nitrate, ask your doctor for advice.

Levitra is not advisable for men with serious heart conditions (such as heart failure) nor men with liver failure or severe kidney disease. Your doctor will be able to advise if you are able to take Levitra.

I am 44 years old with diabetes and now have ED. My doctor says that Levitra might be better for men with diabetes than the other drugs. Is this true?

All three drugs have had research trials conducted in diabetes. Your doctor is correct in saying that, in the Levitra study, more men with diabetes thought that the drug had improved their erections compared with the other two drugs. However, the characteristics of the people in these studies differed quite considerably. This factor could affect the outcome and therefore the results cannot be directly compared at the moment.

What side effects can I expect from Levitra?

Levitra is generally well tolerated, although some men will experience side effects. These are due to effects of Levitra on other parts of the body apart from the penis and the most common ones are headache, facial flushing, indigestion and a stuffy or runny nose. Similar side effects are seen with drugs that act in the same way as Levitra.

Side effects with Levitra are rarely unpleasant enough to make men stop taking it and it is often found that, with continued use, the side effects tend to disappear. If you are bothered by side effects, then you should discuss these with your doctor.

How does Levitra compare with Cialis over Viagra?

In laboratory research conditions, Levitra is the most powerful of the presently available phosphodiesterases (compared with Cialis and Viagra). The question is whether then this equates to a superiority in a 'clinical' setting where healthy and difficult-to-treat groups, such as men with diabetes, are taking it. Up to now there have been no head-to-head data published, so for now we cannot answer the question as to which drug is 'better' or indeed which drug men prefer. At this stage, what can be said confidently is that this is another highly effective drug offering another choice for men with ED.

Can I get Levitra on the NHS?

The NHS has restricted the types of patients with ED who can get treatments paid for by the NHS and this includes Levitra. Your doctor will know whether you come into one of these categories, which are discussed above under Viagra, but generally you have to have some other disease, such as diabetes or spinal cord injury. If this is the case, then, unless you are normally exempt, you will still have to pay a prescription charge for Levitra.

If you are eligible to be prescribed Levitra on the NHS, then your doctor will write the letters 'SLS' (standing for Selected List Scheme) next to the drug name on the prescription. If these letters are not on the prescription, the pharmacist will ask you to pay for Levitra.

You may also be able to get Levitra on the NHS if you are diagnosed as suffering severe distress as a result of your ED. This diagnosis may have to be made by a hospital specialist rather than by your own GP.

The majority of patients have to pay for their ED treatments (although the consultation with the doctor is still free), but a prescription from your doctor is still needed. It is not possible to buy Levitra 'over the counter' from a pharmacist.

Cialis

What doses of Cialis are available in the UK?

There are two doses available: 10 mg (marked with C10)and 20 mg tablets (marked with C20).

How is Cialis different from Viagra?

Cialis and Viagra are in the same class of drugs (they are both PDE5 inhibitors and allow relaxation of the smooth muscle of the penis). They both need sexual stimulation to work. However, they have different chemical structures. One of the main differences is the duration of action of Cialis. Cialis offers a period of responsiveness of 24–36 hours. This will be very important for some men who find it very difficult to estimate accurately when they might have sex. Other men also complain that having to take the tablet immediately before sex makes the situation 'medical'. Clearly a longer window of opportunity could be beneficial for them also. There is no interaction between Cialis and food, whereas Viagra's onset of activity may be delayed by food.

Is Cialis better than Viagra?

There have been no controlled clinical trials comparing men taking the optimum doses of Cialis with Viagra, so a direct comparison cannot be made regarding which drug people prefer. What can be said clearly are that they are both very safe, very effective drugs, and it will up to the patient to decide which is the best for them in a particular social setting.

Can the tablets be split?

The tablets are not designed to be split.

How well does Cialis work?

In a general population study, 81% men stated their erections improved with the 20 mg dose and 75% of attempts for full sexual intercourse were successful. In men with diabetes, 76% reported an improvement in their erections and 58% of attempts for full sexual intercourse were successful. In men taking drugs for high blood pressure, 84% of men reported improvements in their erections.

If Cialis lasts for 24 hours, does this mean erections will last for 24 hours?

No, Cialis is only effective with sexual stimulation. No one has reported episodes of priapism (prolonged erection) when they have used Cialis.

My days are rather hectic and sometimes I have no idea when I am going to have sex with my partner. When should I take Cialis for the best effect?

It can be taken from 30 minutes to 12 hours prior to sexual activity. The effects of Cialis may persist up to 36 hours after you have taken the tablet. This means that you can take the tablet some time before having sex and choose when the time is right for you and your partner.

Will it be OK to take my Cialis tablet while I have my evening meal?

Cialis can be taken with or without food. This is also useful for planning sex.

I am on nitrates for my heart condition. I know that I wasn't allowed Viagra. Can I be prescribed Cialis?

I'm afraid the answer is absolutely no! Cialis must not be used with any form of nitrate. All patients who use currently marketed phosphodiesterase type 5 (PDE5) inhibitors will be advised to avoid the use of nitrates together with Cialis, Viagra or Levitra. Talk to your GP about the many other methods of helping your ED.

Are there any side effects of Cialis and how do they compare to Viagra's?

There are no head-to-head data comparing Cialis and Viagra. However, most of the side effects that are seen with Cialis are what would be expected from a PDE5 inhibitor. These are headache, facial flushing and dyspepsia. Unlike the other PDE5 inhibitors Cialis can also lead to back pain and muscle ache, but there can be visual side effects as with the other PDE5 inhibitors. These side effects were also seen in original Viagra studies when men were taking Viagra every day. They are thought to be associated with the longer duration of action of Cialis. The reason that they occur is not known. They are mild and relieved by movement or stretching. The amount of men stopping treatment because of these side effects is extremely low. The side effects are usually mild to moderate in nature and lessen with repeated or reduced dosing.

So far, having Cialis in the system for a longer time has not caused problems, but further research is ongoing. Some research is suggesting that this type of drug might protect the heart, and therefore having a longer-acting drug could be more beneficial for your cardiovascular system.

Has Cialis any advantages over Viagra or Levitra?

The main advantage with Cialis is that it has a long 'half-life' – what this means is that the drug will be effective for longer than Viagra or Levitra, so you won't have to have sex soon after taking it, taking the pressure off planning intercourse precisely. This can be a major advantage to some people, particularly those not in a regular relationship, who feel at present that they are at risk of wasting their Viagra tablet if they take it and then don't have sex in the ensuing few hours. It will also be advantageous to those people who feel that taking a tablet immediately before sex 'medicalizes' the whole situation.

Another advantage is that, unlike Viagra, the absorption of Cialis does not appear to be affected by food. This means that it will work just as well when taken after a meal.

Do you think that Cialis will be better than Viagra in the long term?

At the moment, this is not possible to say. It is dangerous to try to compare the results of studies between Viagra and Cialis, as the trials have been made in different people, or were carried out or assessed differently. For the future, you might be offered a selection of these tablets, so that you can take some of each to see which suits you best, or indeed have some of each to take in different social circumstances.

Apomorphine (Uprima)

In 2001 a tablet called Uprima was launched. The chemical name for this drug is apomorphine. It is distantly related to morphine, but has none of its addictive properties. About 70% of men who get erections with Uprima have an erection within 20 minutes. It is important to remember that to help Uprima work (the same as for Viagra), you need to have some sexual foreplay to get yourself aroused. Some of its characteristics are listed in the box opposite.

There is a caution on the packaging of this drug for men with heart problems taking nitrates with Uprima. This relates to an early study where patients took high doses of apomorphine and nitrates were taken together, and people had a significant fall in their blood pressure. However, at the doses that have been licensed, there does not appear to be any sort of clinically worrying interactions.

How does apomorphine work?

In the brain, when there is sexual stimulation, a variety of chemicals are produced, which eventually lead to an erection. One of these chemicals is called dopamine, and apomorphine works by stimulating the central dopamine receptors and thus making the brain think that there is an increase in dopamine. Therefore, the body's response to sexual stimulation is increased.

Advantages and disadvantages of apomorphine

Advantages

- It acts faster than other oral tablets.
- Unlike Viagra, absorption of this drug is not affected by food.
- There are no specific safety problems for older men taking Uprima.
- Side effects are usually mild.

Disadvantages

- It shouldn't be used with similar drugs used to treat illnesses such as Parkinson's disease.
- If you have liver or kidney failure, you should discuss with your doctor whether you should have apomorphine.
- It does not work for as many men as Viagra, Cialis, Levitra or injection therapy.

Do I take Uprima in the same way that I take Viagra?

No, Uprima is placed under your tongue, where it dissolves in about 10–15 minutes. It is made in two doses, 2 mg and 3 mg, and the tablets for these two doses look quite different. The 2 mg tablets have five sides and the 3 mg tablets have three sides. Because it is put under the tongue, Uprima works faster than swallowed tablets do.

Does Uprima work for everyone?

No. No tablets will work for everybody. Research into Uprima showed that, with the 3 mg dosage, erections were firm enough for intercourse approximately half the time, as assessed by both men and their partners.

I have been prescribed Uprima. Is it as safe as Viagra?

Most men have not had problems in the studies done so far. The most common side effects have been nausea, yawning, dizziness and headache, which were mild and did not last long enough to stop men from wanting to carry on with these studies. Some men fainted who were taking higher doses of Uprima than had been licensed for usage, but with the 2 mg and 3 mg dosages, only 0.2% men fainted (that is only 2 per 1000). Before fainting, you would tend to feel nauseous, sweaty and light-headed. If you take the drug and feel these symptoms come on, you should stop sexual activity and lie down. So long as you don't take more than you have been prescribed, you should not have any problems.

Can I take Uprima and Viagra together?

This is an interesting question, because it is one that many doctors have thought about. They seem to think it would be possible because the drugs have different ways of working and have different side-effects, but there have been no clinical trials so far so it **cannot** be recommended at this stage.

8
Alprostadil treatment

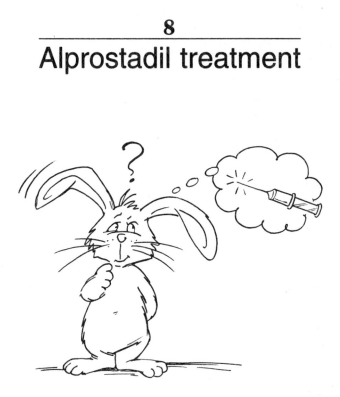

If oral treatment doesn't work for you, then there are other choices open to you and we discuss these in the next three chapters. Treatment with a drug called alprostadil is either by injection into your penis (Caverject dual chamber/vials, Viridal duo) or through your urethra (where you urinate from) using the MUSE system, and these can be effective alternative treatments for some men. Alprostadil is a form of a natural substance in your body, technically known as prostaglandin E1, which opens up blood vessels. It is effective in men with a wide range of medical disorders (including diabetes), heart disease, surgery and injury (such as damage to the spinal cord or pelvis).

For the future, alprostadil is being developed as a cream to rub into the skin (see later section in this chapter).

Caverject dual chamber/vials and Viridal duo injections

Devices to inject alprostadil (Caverject dual chamber/vials and Viridal duo) use a very small needle but injecting yourself is not very painful. Both come in a dual-chamber preparation (see Figure 8.1), which makes preparing and administering the drug a lot simpler. The drug and the water in which it dissolves are now

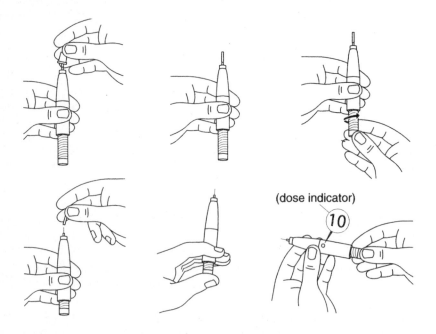

Figure 8.1 Preparation of Caverject.

in the same syringe. Previously they were in different containers, which made the mixing process more complicated, but now it is very simple.

Is Caverject dual chamber/vials different from alprostadil?

Caverject dual chamber/vials is an alprostadil-based injection therapy. The name 'Caverject' is just the registered pharmaceutical brand name of this alprostadil-based therapy.

Is alprostadil suitable for everybody with ED?

Unfortunately not. Men with or at risk of blood clots or who are using blood thinners, such as heparin or warfarin, should not use it. It is not appropriate for men with penile implants, or men whose impotence is due to leakage in the blood vessels. There are also side effects (see question below).

I have tried Viagra unsuccessfully, which was gutting. On the other hand, the injection treatment sounds frightening as I'm a real baby having injections. What is 'Caverject dual chamber/vials' exactly?

Caverject dual chamber/vials (alprostadil) is a vasoactive drug. This means that when it is injected into the penis it will cause the blood vessels to relax and increase the blood flow. This is referred to as an intracavernosal injection, and it helps to produce an erection (see Figure 1.1). It is a very effective treatment for ED, producing stronger and more predictable erections than other treatments.

It is particularly useful if tablets have not been successful, or if you want to know whether your ED is caused by a reduced blood flow in your case. Intracavernosal therapy is easy to use. However, the need for an injection means that having sex might not be spontaneous, so it is not ideal for everyone.

Alprostadil is the most frequently prescribed drug that helps to fill your penis with blood. Following the first injection, you might get improvement in your erections, as if your mechanism has 'woken-up'!

I've been really depressed since I've been unable to have an erection, so I'm prepared to try Caverject dual chamber/vials. Will anyone teach me how to administer the injections?

Yes. your nurse or doctor will administer your first injection, or they will talk you through it, and then observe you injecting yourself. The injections are very simple to prepare now as they

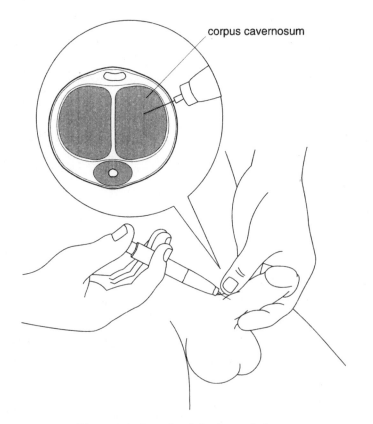

corpus cavernosum

Figure 8.2 Caverject injection technique.

come in a dual-chamber preparation (see Figure 8.1). Figure 8.2 shows you how to do the injection (see also Figure 1.1 for full anatomy details.

While sitting down, hold the tip of your penis between your left thumb and forefinger (if you are right-handed) and gently squeeze. The injection site will then bulge out – make sure the foreskin is stretched.

Hold the needle and syringe in your right hand at right angles to the penis. Inject into the shaft of the penis, near the base, away from the middle and avoiding any visible veins. It is important that the injections are given into the side of the penis. At the bottom of the penis, as you are looking at it, is the tube called the urethra through which the urine and semen flow, and on the very top are where the nerves and blood vessels lie. Clearly, both of these areas need to be avoided. Push the needle all the way into the bulgy part ensuring that the syringe is held at a right angle to the penis. Once the needle has been inserted into the penis, inject the fluid. Once all the fluid has been injected, pull the needle out of the penis. Press gently on the needle mark and massage the penis, this will help the alprostadil spread through the penis.

Do not inject into the tip of the penis (glans head) as this will be extremely painful but, more importantly, you will not obtain an erection because you haven't injected the part of the penis where the blood is stored during erections (corpora cavernosa – see Figure 1.1).

If any bruising or bleeding occurs, check with your doctor that you are injecting correctly.

I'm prepared to have a go, but keep thinking that it isn't the ideal preparation for making love and not at all romantic! Does the injection hurt?

The needle is small, so the injection is not usually painful. A burning pain from the drug itself occurs only in a small percentage of men, but once you have used injections a few times you will find the burning sensation will subside.

My partner and I normally go clubbing on Saturdays and I don't think it would be suitable to take needles and things with us, in case the club owners think we're drug addicts! Should I inject before we go out? How long does the erection last after I have administered the injection?

The erection following an injection may last for 1–2 hours. Once you have ejaculated, the penis usually starts to become soft (flaccid) within minutes. If your erection last longer than 4 hours, your penis could be damaged, so it would be advisable to go to your local A&E Department for aspiration to relieve the erection.

Am I going to do myself damage if I have sex every day now? How often can I use injections?

You should only inject once every 24 hours but you can have up to three injections per week. Remember to alternate the injection site slightly each time that you inject, to reduce the risk of scarring.

Once you can get over 'needle phobia' this sounds ideal but, if it's such a good idea, why do men stop using injection therapy?

In spite of its general success, self-injection therapy has a high dropout rate. There are various reasons why men stop using injections:

- They get bored with having to inject themselves.
- They don't actually like the injecting business.
- They decide to try other treatments.
- Their erections have got better.
- They have side effects from alprostadil.
- Their partner objects to use of injections.
- Their relationship has broken up.

I'm worried I'm doing my penis harm, though I like the feeling of being hard again, but I keep getting a burning sensation where I do the injections. Should I stop?

Alprostadil does have some side effects – these include burning and pain at the injection site. To help prevent this side effect, you could try a lower starting dose increasing with subsequent doses until you get an erection. If you are not already using a dual-chamber preparation it may be worthwhile changing to one, because fewer men complain about 'stinging' or 'burning' when they use a dual-chamber preparation rather than a vial.

I have quite low blood pressure normally, and after an injection get faint. Is this to do with my low blood pressure?

Sudden low blood pressure can occur in some men. Symptoms include dizziness, light-headedness and fainting. If you are getting these symptoms, lie down immediately and raise your legs.

Sex is now wonderful with my partner and she would like me to do it more often! However, I get a lot of bruising where I inject myself. Should this happen?

Bruising (or bleeding) usually happens when you haven't injected properly and you have either injected into a vein or have caught a vein with the needle. Figure 8.2 shows you how to do this, or look at the patient information leaflet inside the pack. Check with your doctor or nurse if you are still unsure whether you are doing the injection properly.

The last time I used alprostadil, I had a really long erection, which actually was quite painful. Is this common?

No, this is not common; fewer than 1% of men will suffer from this. If you follow the instructions given by the nurse or doctor who has taught you how to inject, then you will have only a low risk of having a prolonged erection. This is called priapism (prolonged erection – see question in Chapter 1) and is a side effect of alprostadil. If it occurs again, apply a cold flannel or ice wrapped in a cloth for 10-minute periods to your inner thigh; this may help to reduce the blood flow, or try going for a brisk walk. Cough medicine containing Sudafed will also help to reduce the blood flow in the penis. Some men have found that, if they ejaculate while they have a prolonged erection, this has helped the penis to become flaccid (soft); if the prolonged erection is painful, do not try to ejaculate. If the erection lasts more than 4 hours, go to the local clinic or casualty immediately, taking with you the treatment that you have used and tell them when you last used it. The situation is easily fixed by a doctor who will take some of the blood out of the penis. Most prolonged erections resolve themselves with no treatment needed.

Before you use alprostadil again, you should talk to your doctor or nurse who taught you, in case you need to reduce the dose of alprostadil.

I have used injections for over a year now, but find that I have a hard patch of skin where I usually inject myself. Should I stop doing it?

No, but it is advisable to get your doctor to look at it. Scarring of the penis at the injection site is a possible side effect, but it is rare and usually causes no long-term problems. You could try alternating injections on each side of your penis.

I like the idea of injections, but alprostadil doesn't work for me. Are there any other types of injections?

Until the introduction of alprostadil, the two drugs used for injection therapy had been papaverine and phentolamine. Side effects of these two therapies are usually minor but include pain, ulcers, and prolonged erections (priapism), which sometimes require using a needle to withdraw blood or another drug to reverse the process.

How much do Caverject dual chamber/vials cost and can they be obtained on the NHS?

If your ED is being caused by illnesses or diseases that are not listed in Schedule 11 (i.e. if you have to have a private prescription for ED treatment regardless of what the treatment choice is – see Chapter 5), we would recommended 'phoning around different chemists/pharmacies to see how much they charge for a private prescription. You will be surprised at how much they vary in price!

All ED therapies are available only on prescription. The cause of your impotence will determine whether or not you can obtain a NHS prescription or if you will need a private prescription.

My GP is a lady and I am a bit embarrassed about talking about my problems to her. Can I get Caverject dual chamber/vials anywhere else such as a private clinic?

We can appreciate you may find it embarrassing seeing a female doctor, but you may only need to see her once if she is willing to write a repeat prescription for you. If you have already been assessed for your impotence, then the doctor who has assessed you has probably written to your GP, so she will be aware of your condition. Would you avoid going to see your GP for another illness fearing that she say may ask you about how you are coping with the injection therapy? If this is the case, then you should consider changing to another practice.

You can attend a private clinic for an ED assessment but some private doctors would request a referral letter from your GP before seeing you. If you have to attend a private clinic on a regular basis in order to obtain a prescription, this could work out to be expensive, especially if you are entitled to treatment on the NHS!

Injection treatment sounds ideal for me, but I'm often away on business. Can my wife be given the prescription for Caverject dual chamber on my behalf when I can't see the doctor myself?

If you have already been assessed and started injection therapy, then you could ask your GP if you could have a repeat prescription for Caverject dual chamber/vials, and your wife would be able to collect it. However, if you have never been assessed or haven't been taught how to use Caverject dual chamber/vials, then ethically the doctor could not prescribe the injections for you.

I've been using Caverject dual chamber for some time now, but it doesn't seem to be working any more. Will I need a higher dose?

As you get older, you may find that the effect of intracavernosal therapy is gradually lost. If you have already been instructed on how to adjust your Caverject dual chamber/vials dose, then you will be able to increase the dose. You should talk to your doctor or nurse about the reduced effect Caverject dual chamber/vials is having, in case you are not injecting properly.

I have been using injection therapy for 5 years and can feel lumps on the side of my penis. What are they?

These are caused by 'fibrosis' – this is a thickening of the erectile tissue – which may occur after using intracavernosal therapy for some time. If this happens, stop injecting immediately and consult your doctor.

I have had MS for many years. Could intracavernosal injections help me, as I find getting an erection quite difficult these days?

Yes, injections are particularly useful when there is damage to the nervous system. As long as you don't use any blood thinning medication, such as heparin or warfarin, there is no reason as to why this would not work for you.

Patients with nerve damage causing ED tend to require a lower dose of alprostadil, so your GP will be careful when establishing the correct dose for you.

Some years ago I had a road accident and am now in a wheelchair. Do you think I could learn how to use Caverject dual chamber?

Yes. You will have similar problems to people with MS, and many men with paraplegia (where they have lost sensation in the legs and trunk) find that these injections are a very good form of treatment. The same caution applies as in the question above, in that many such men are young (and thus have 'young' blood vessels) so you will react to relatively small doses of alprostadil.

I use alprostadil injections and have noticed that, when my penis is erect, it is no longer straight, but bends towards the right. Is this normal?

When intracavernosal injections are used regularly, they may damage the penile tissue; scarring of the penis (Peyronie's disease) then develops causing the penis to bend (see Chapter 12). Scarring occurs in about 1 in 12 men who have used injection therapy for more than a year. You must stop using the treatment until you have seen your GP; you can start injecting again when the condition has been sorted out.

I became impotent following a back operation. I haven't been able to use Viagra. Could Caverject dual chamber help me?

Intracavernosal therapy is particularly useful for ED from damage to the nervous system, which sounds like what happened to you as a result of surgery, so theoretically yes it could. You should visit your GP for assessment and advice.

Since I was diagnosed with Parkinson's, I am unable to inject myself. Could my wife be taught how to do it?

If you have an unsteady hand because of multiple sclerosis, Parkinson's disease or stroke, then a willing partner can be taught to inject. If you are overweight and have difficulty seeing where to inject or have poor eyesight, then again a willing partner could be very useful!

MUSE

MUSE is an acronym for Medicated Urethral System for Erection. MUSE uses the same drug (alprostadil) as goes into the penis with the intracavernosal injections.

Rather than the drug being injected, it is inserted directly into the urethra (the tube that the urine and semen come through) via a plastic tube and in the form of a small pellet. Once it is in the urethra, the drug then dissolves and is absorbed into the penile tissue.

In order to help the drug absorb into your penis, you will be asked to pass urine immediately before inserting the pellet as this lubricates the urethra and eases insertion and also stops the possibility of you needing to urinate immediately afterwards and hence possibly washing it out. The advantages and disadvantages of MUSE are listed in the box.

I am using MUSE, but it does not seem to be working. Why is this?

As stated in the box, MUSE is only effective in only about one-third of men, so unfortunately you are probably one of the two-thirds where MUSE does not work properly!

Most men will have opted for tablets originally, and will have progressed on to MUSE if these failed. If this is the position you find yourself in, then it may be worthwhile returning to your GP to talk about the newer treatment options that are now available

---

Features of MUSE

Advantages

- There are no needles involved and so it is suitable for people with a needle phobia, particularly about injections into the penis.
- It is a method suitable for people who have poor eyesight and/or limited manual dexterity, e.g. those with severe arthritis in their hands.
- There is a lower risk of prolonged erections than with injections.

Disdvantages

- It is effective in only about a third to a half of patients using it.
- The effect is slower to start, compared with intracavernosal injections.
- A significant number of men will experience pain in their penises, which is related not only to the insertion of the pellet, but also to the absorption of the drug in the urethra, because about 50 times more drug needs to be applied as compared with injection therapy.

---

as tablets, which may not have been available when you first started to use MUSE.

If you are one of those patients who could not take Viagra because you were also taking some specific sorts of heart tablets, again, there are now newer tablets that do not have this restriction, so it may be worthwhile returning to your doctor to talk about these.

If you chose to try MUSE without trying other treatment options, and it is now not working for you, again, get some information on other treatments such as tablets or injections.

If you are one of the very few unfortunate men for whom therapies such as tablets, injections and MUSE have not worked, then it would be well worth trying a vacuum therapy device (see Chapter 9), which is a very safe alternative and has a 90% success rate.

I am gay and my partner and I have oral sex. Is it safe to use MUSE and have oral sex?

There has been no research done in this area. If your partner has oral sex with you before the pellet is absorbed (which will be less than 5 minutes) and you do not use a condom, the pellet may become dislodged from your urethra and thus be ineffective.

If you have oral sex after you have an erection, then there should be no danger to your partner of having sex without a condom (indeed there is a significant amount of prostaglandin in the ejaculate anyway, so the addition from MUSE will not make any difference). The manufacturers of MUSE advise people to use a condom, however, to be on the safe side.

The information leaflet tells me to store MUSE in a fridge. How long can I leave MUSE out of the fridge before using it?

Unopened pouches of MUSE should be kept in a refrigerator at 2–8°C. MUSE will be more effective if you allow it to warm to room temperature before use, as this will make it more comfortable to insert and also aid its absorption. MUSE can be stored at room temperature (below 30°C) for up to 14 days.

If MUSE has been out of the fridge for 3 days and then put back into the fridge, the 'clock stops' until it is taken out of the fridge again.

I was given MUSE first while I was in hospital. It worked then, but now it doesn't. Why is this?

The original studies of MUSE showed that it worked in a hospital or a clinic in about two-thirds of men, but even of this group, only two-thirds were successful at home. This could have many reasons:

- not using the insertion technique properly
- not allowing time for the erection to develop

- psychological causes associated with erectile failure as listed in Chapter 2
- the disease process that has caused your ED progressing since you used the medication in hospital
- you or your partner being very anxious about using this at home, stopping the medication working.

I used to use injections, but wanted to have sex more often than the recommended frequency, so I'm trying MUSE. How often can I use this method?

You will probably need to use one tube each time you wish to achieve an erection. However, the company who make MUSE suggest that you do not use more than two tubes in any 24-hour period and not more than seven applicators in any 7-day period.

Following a car accident I am now classified as a quadriplegic, even though I have some use of my hands. I have also been impotent since the accident and have tried both Uprima and Viagra with poor results. I would like to try Caverject but I am unable to inject. Is there any other way I can take alprostadil?

Instead of injecting alprostadil, you can insert a small wax pellet into your urethra (water pipe). If you have a urinary urethral catheter you may not be suitable to use MUSE, so it is advisable to get your GP to refer you to see a specialist.

MUSE isn't as effective as Caverject, so you might need to revert to using injections. Do not despair if you are not able to inject yourself with Caverject – your sexual partner can be trained to do it as long as both you and your partner are happy with that arrangement.

I've not found any other pill or injection suitable for me and am very keen that MUSE does work. Are there any practical hints on how to make MUSE more effective?

Yes there are:

- Urinate before you insert MUSE as this helps both to lubricate the urethra and to dissolve the pellet.
- Insert the applicator all the way up to the collar.
- Keep MUSE in position up to the collar for 5 seconds.
- Massage your penis after insertion – this helps to dissolve the pellet.
- Stand or walk around for 10 minutes after administration.
- Follow the storage recommendations and take MUSE out of the refrigerator and warm it up prior to use.
- Use barrier protection if your partner is pregnant. or at risk of getting pregnant.
- Do not touch the tube stem or tip as this will contaminate it.
- Do not apply any additional lubrication, e.g. K-Y Jelly, as this may prevent MUSE from working.
- Do not push in or pull out the applicator button before use or you will lose the pellet.
- Do not insert MUSE while you are lying down, or lie down as you are inserting it, as this may prevent it from working properly.

Talk to your doctor or nurse if you experience problems.

MUSE has not worked for me and neither has Viagra. Can I use them both together?

Many people have asked this question. It is an appealing idea in that the Viagra tablets and MUSE will work in different ways and therefore taking a combination could be good. However, there have been no studies so far into how effective this combination might be, nor to explore its possible harmful effects; therefore for the present, combination of these two therapies **cannot** be recommended.

The future

There is much research being done in the area of sexual function and perhaps in the future men will be offered a combination of tablets as suggested in Chapter 7 or a cream in order to tackle the problem in different ways.

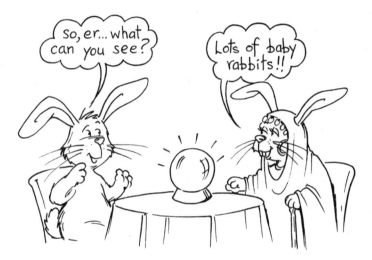

Creams

Are there any creams on the market yet?

To date, medications delivered topically (through skin patches, ointments or sprays) have not been very successful, but research is ongoing for drugs that can be applied to the skin of the penis rather than given by injections or taken by mouth.

- In one study, 30% of men using a cream containing prostaglandin E2 had erections.

- In China there is a cream called Alprox TD that is applied directly to the penis. It contains the same medication (prostaglandin E1) as is given at present by injection into the penis. The results of the trials from Asia and America look promising, but it will be some years before this medication is available in Europe. Trials are also ongoing here in the UK. The cream is applied to the tip of penis 15 minutes before intercourse. Many men would prefer to use a cream and you should ask your doctor whether it is available yet, if you would like to try it.

• A tanning lotion called Melanotan II is showing promise in trials, but men with heart problems should probably not take this medication.

• An Egyptian study reported that a cream made of aminophylline, isosorbide dinitrate and ergot alkaloids helped towards full erection in 58% of men with impotence caused by a number of disorders, and in 82% of men where the disorder had a psychological basis.

• There is also an aerosol spray made from minoxidil, a drug that relaxes smooth muscles and helps open up blood vessels – this helped 25% of a very small group of men where ED had been caused by spinal cord injury. It is not as effective as vacuum devices or injections, but it is easier to use and will be worth more research.

9

Vacuum therapy devices (VTD)

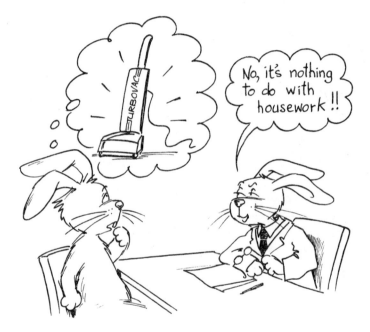

Vacuum devices are an effective treatment for ED suitable for most men. A VTD consists of a vacuum chamber with a 'constriction' ring, and a hand or battery-operated pump. They work by creating a negative pressure around your penis, increasing the blood flow, thus inducing an erection. To be able to maintain your erection, a constriction ring needs to be applied to the base of your penis (Figure 9.1). The rings are made either from latex/rubber or silicon depending on the manufacturer, and in various sizes.

Advantages and disadvantages are listed in the box.

Features of VTDs

Advantages

- If you have to pay for private prescriptions for your treatment, over time the VTD can work out cheaper than other prescriptions, as it will last for years, although the constriction rings will need to be replaced.
- There are no needles involved.
- They are available on prescription.
- VTDs can be used many times a day, if required!

Disadvantages

- VTDs can remove the spontaneity from sexual relations.
- They can be fiddly and a bit unsightly, but with continued use, they do become easier to put on.
- The penis will be enlarged and rigid, but may not stand erect, as with a natural erection, so that you may have to try alternative sexual positions with your partner.
- Ejaculation can be delayed or absent.
- If the constriction ring is left on too long, it can cause damage to the tissues of your penis by blocking off the blood supply.
- Partners sometimes complain about the penis feeling cold.

I'm thrilled with my VTD and my partner thinks it is the business! How often can I use it?

As often as you want to, as long as you give the penis time for the blood flow to return to normal. It is normally recommended that you have an hour's break between using the constriction ring and the ring doesn't stay on your penis for more than 30 minutes each time.

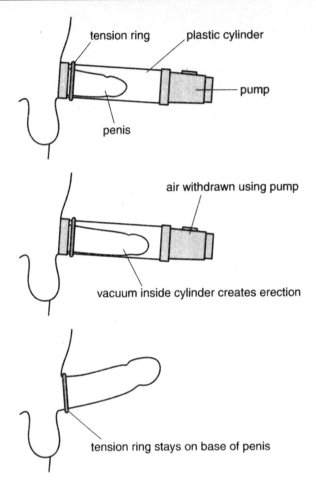

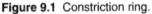

Figure 9.1 Constriction ring.

At the moment I am using MUSE, which is so-so. Would I get an even better erection if I used a VTD as well?

There has been some research into the use of MUSE and VTDs together. This has shown that VTDs can increase the effectiveness of MUSE but, before using this combination of treatments, discuss it first with the doctor who prescribes your MUSE.

I am going to try a VTD as my first treatment for ED. Is it going to work for me?

VTDs are an effective treatment for ED and it is one of the most successful; unfortunately the VTD is not suitable for everybody. Men who use anticoagulants such as warfarin and heparin should talk to their GP before using them, as VTDs can cause bleeding and bruises. Men with tight or scarred foreskins might find the skin splits because of the negative pressure created.

I like using the pump, but don't want to use a condom as well. Will the constriction ring act as a form of birth control?

No. The constriction ring can reduce the amount of ejaculate when you orgasm but there is no guarantee that it will stop all your sperm and semen from entering your partner.

Have you got any tips for using a VTD?

These tips have come from a user so we hope you will find them useful:

- When you first get the VTD, practise using it twice a day for 7 days before using it for proper sexual intercourse
- Refer to the 'release pressure button' if, during pumping up your erection, the constriction becomes too tight. Release off, rest and start again.
- Use plenty of something like K-Y Jelly round the base of your penis and the base of the tube to create a good vacuum for a hard erection.
- Stroke the base of the 'internal penis' from your anus to the scrotum to help increase blood supply into the 'outer penis'.

Are VTDs available on the NHS?

Since April 2002 VTDs are now included in Schedule 11. They are supplied with instructions and a video. Many sexual health clinics will be able to lend you the equipment to try first before you get one or will be able to demonstrate how to use one. For up-to-date information on VTDs you can phone the Sexual Dysfunction Association (formerly the Impotence Association) – see Appendix 1 – or speak to your doctor or nurse.

When I went to buy a VTD, I discovered that there are different sizes on offer. How do I select the right sized constriction ring for me?

When you buy a VTD, there are indeed a selection of different sizes of constriction rings. It is a bit of trial and error to start with, although some manufacturers supply a measurer, but the general rule is to start by using the middle size ring. If you find that you can maintain an erection with this size but it is too uncomfortable, then you need to increase the size of ring; but, if you find that you can't maintain the erection, then the ring is too big, and you need to try a smaller one.

Occasionally some men need to use two constriction rings, but this is unusual.

Do these rings last forever, or do they have to be replaced?

The ring will become worn and lose its elasticity in time – then you may find that you can't maintain your erection and you should replace it. You'll have lots of warning, so replacing it will be no problem.

I am unable to ejaculate when using the pump. Why is this?

Your orgasm will be normal, but your ejaculate (sperm and semen) can get trapped behind the constriction ring. A VTD is therefore not suitable if you are trying to get your partner pregnant! There is no need to worry if you don't ejaculate because the semen will seep out when the ring is removed or when you next pass urine.There is a pump on the market (Owen Mumford – see Appendix 1) which has rings and loops to pull to one side at the point of ejaculation so that the sperm does not get trapped.

I normally make love in the 'missionary position'. My wife is a bit straight-laced (she's 7 years older than me) and she's not even that keen on me using a VTD. Do I have to learn new tricks?!

This is, of course, down to individual preference; however, many people find the device more successful if they use it either standing or sitting. This is a good opportunity to discuss different positions with your partner. You might 'inject' some new excitement into your lovemaking!

The success of a VTD actually relies heavily on partner involvement. Men in long-term relationships with understanding partners will benefit most from VTDs.

There seem to be quite a few side effects with the other treatments that I have tried. Are there any with a VTD?

VTDs have very few side effects other than bruising, and are therefore a safe treatment option.

Partners have sometimes complained of the penis feeling cold. The constriction ring does reduce the blood flow out of the penis, so blood can't get back in once the VTD has been applied. This can cause the penis to become mottled in colour and feel cold. Once the constriction ring has been removed, normal warmth and colour of the penis returns. You also might not be able to ejaculate when you have an orgasm. This is primarily due to the constriction ring but it is nothing to worry about.

I have just bought a VTD. I must say it doesn't seem my thing at all and I'm rather concerned at my partner's likely reaction. Will I get an erection quickly once it is on?

VTD produces a satisfactory erection in most patients in less than 10 minutes. It may take longer when you first start to use a VTD, as you have to overcome several hurdles – these include how to use it, embarrassment and a possible reduction in foreplay.

It's so unsexy, planning sex like a railway timetable. Supposing my partner and I don't make love immediately? How long can I keep the constriction ring on for?

The constriction ring must be removed after 30 minutes to prevent damage to the tissues (called 'ischaemia') in the penis. The good thing is that, unlike other treatments, your erection should be immediate and last for half an hour.

I have tried using a VTD and find it useless and a waste of money. I might as well chuck it away.

Don't give up! Sometimes a VTD does not work because the 'airtight seal' at the base of the penis has not been created while you are using it, and so you are unable to create a negative pressure.

Another reason is that you might not have an adequate blood flow to the penis (usually because of blocked arteries) for a VTD to create a negative pressure.

Finally, if you suffer from Peyronie's disease (curvature of the penis when erect – see Chapter 12), then you could find a VTD uncomfortable. There are lot of other treatments you could use instead, so don't give up at this first hurdle!

My girlfriend told me that I could get the same effect as the VTD from putting my penis into a bottle once it was hard. Is she right?

Do not attempt to do this! Your erection will remain until the bottle has been broken off and this in itself is a very dangerous thing to have to do and could cause further damage.

10
Surgery for ED

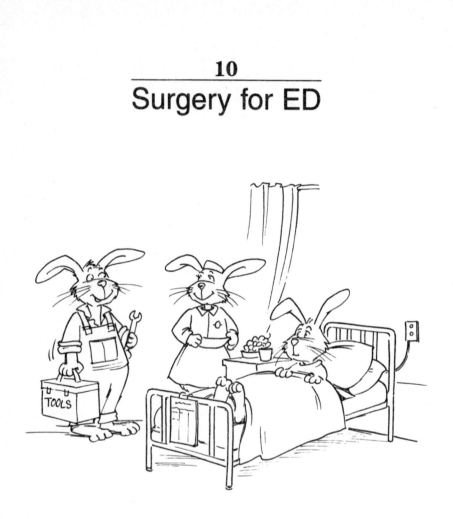

Your doctor might have suggested that you have an operation for your ED for one of two major reasons. Firstly, you might need surgery to correct abnormalities in your blood vessels or you might benefit from a prosthesis for your penis. Both these operations are discussed here.

Vascular surgery

I had to have heart surgery some time ago and now cannot get a good erection. I have tried Viagra and also the vacuum pump, but neither were really successful. Would surgery help me?

If your impotence is caused by damage to the arteries or blood vessels (and this may well be the reason if you have already had heart surgery), vascular surgery might be an option. Two types of operations are available: revascularization (or bypass) surgery and venous ligation.

In **revascularization** an artery is taken from your leg and then surgically connected to the arteries at the back of your penis, bypassing the blockages and restoring blood flow. Young men with local sites of arterial blockage generally achieve the best results. In some studies improvement in ED was seen in 50–75% of men after 5 years.

An operation on your arteries sounds a very good idea. After all, if there is a problem getting blood into your penis, then repairing those arteries would seem the best way forward. However, the reality is not as rosy, as the real long-term benefits from this surgery have not been good, probably because the blood vessels become affected by the same disease processes that have blocked the original vessels.

Venous ligation is performed when your penis is unable to store a sufficient amount of blood to maintain an erection (venous leakage syndrome). This operation, which was fashionable for many years, ties off or removes veins that are causing an excessive amount of blood to drain from your erection chambers. Success rate is estimated at between 40% and 50% initially, but drops to 15% over the long term. Unless patients are very carefully selected, the long-term success rates from this sort of surgery are obviously not high. It is, of course, important to find a surgeon experienced in this surgery.

Prostheses

A penile prosthesis involves surgery to insert an artificial rod into the penis. It is the final option when all other ED treatments have failed. A prosthesis may benefit men with fibrosis (thickening) following intracavernosal therapy (see Chapter 8), Peyronie's disease (a fibrous plaque or scarring that causes the penis to bend – see Chapter 12) or an untreated prolonged erection (priapism – see Chapters 1 and 2).

My doctor has told me all about prostheses but I didn't realise that there were different types. Which would be best for me?

Three types of prostheses are available: semi-rigid malleable rods, inflatable cylinders and multipart inflatable prostheses, and your doctor has probably already discussed these choices with you. The semirigid rod protrudes and may be embarrassing, while an inflatable three-piece is expensive, but can be pumped up and down. It is important to understand that a prosthesis can never fully replace the erection you might have had when you were younger.

Nowadays a penile prosthesis consists of two rods inserted inside the shaft of your penis and, depending on what sort of rods are chosen, this will either give a permanent erection or an erection as required. The newer types of prostheses, which give an erection as required, have a pump placed inside the scrotum. These inflatable devices give a more acceptable appearance to the penis and are certainly preferable for younger men. However, they are considerably more expensive and also difficult to insert when there is significant scarring in the penis. The advantages and disadvantages of prostheses are listed in the box.

Features of prostheses

Advantages
- They are successful for the vast majority of men.
- They offer long-lasting results.
- They are useful in patients who have Peyronie's disease as well as ED.

Disadvantages
- You can't use treatments like Viagra at the same time.
- They are very expensive.
- Pain can persist for a considerable period of time after the operation.
- Having a prosthesis will not make your sex drive greater; it is just a mechanical means of enabling an erection, and therefore having sex.
- Your penis might seem (to you) to be shorter than you thought.
- You might get less feeling in your penis.
- Some men find that ejaculation is either difficult or not possible for several weeks after the operation.
- If you have a semirigid device, your penis will not get bigger when you have an erection.

I'm absolutely terrified that I can't go back, so before I go ahead with surgery, I'd like to know whether there are any complications from the operation that could cause problems?

Yes there are.

- **Problems during surgery**. If the surgeon finds it difficult to put the cylinders inside your penis, your penis or movement of the cylinders could be damaged; this can result in the so-called 'Concorde' deformity, where the glans lacks support and curves downwards, making penetration awkward.

- **Pain**. This has occurred with the semirigid devices. If pain persists, this may be due to too large cylinders having been fitted. Usually the pain disappears over time, but a very small number of men might need another operation.

- **Infection**. Infection occurs in about 1–10% of operations, and the risk appears to be higher for the newer inflatable devices. Infection can usually be treated with antibiotics, but in severe cases it may mean that the cylinders need to be removed. Insertion requires a general or local anaesthetic. Antibiotics are given during the operation, and this will help to reduce your chances of infection. This can be a major problem for men with diabetes.

- **Erosion of tissues**. Erosion is often associated with infections and can also be due to a cylinder having been inserted for too long. This could result in the cylinder protruding through the skin at the end of your penis. This would need a further operation to remove the cylinders and correct the problem.

- **Mechanical failure**. This is rare but can occur in the pump or the cylinder in the inflatable prostheses. The commonest problem is a scrotal pump riding up too high. This would also need a further operation to remove the cylinders and correct the problem.

It sounds like there are a lot of complications. Are people happy with the results?

In general, the answer to your question is yes. Research shows that most men and their partners are happy following the fitting of their prostheses.

I have had diabetes since I was 38 and my sex life is poor. I wonder what my best option would be. Would a prostheses be suitable for me?

Occasionally, infection can occur when a prosthesis is inserted and infection can lead to failure of the prostheses. Failure occurs more often in people with diabetes or whose immune system is depressed for some reason. You should make sure that your diabetes is kept under strict control and this will help reduce the chances of infection.

I had the operation 3 weeks ago and I still feel very sore. How soon can I have intercourse?

The operation is uncomfortable, and it can take up to 4 weeks for this to settle. You will be taught how to pump an inflatable prosthesis at 4 weeks, and this is when you will be able to have sexual intercourse.

Does my partner have to agree to the operation?

Although it is you who has to undergo surgery, you should talk to your partner or wife before deciding on a penile prosthesis, as she or he will be involved in the future. It will be best for both of you to agree to the procedure together.

I underwent this post-radical prostatectomy 6 months ago. I get no erections and nothing helps. Will things get better naturally or do I need some help?

If you have tried all the treatment options – oral, injection, MUSE and vacuum therapy – then you need to be referred to a urology specialist to discuss a prosthesis. This procedure should not be done until all other options have been tried.

11
Problems with ejaculation

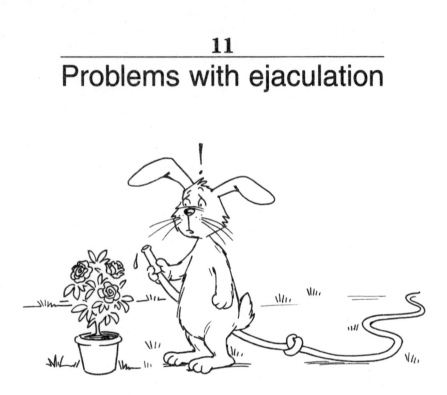

Approximately 40% of men attending sexual dysfunction clinics have problems with ejaculation rather than difficulty having erections: either ejaculating too quickly or not being able to ejaculate at all.

I am confused about what is ejaculation and what is an orgasm. Aren't the two the same thing?

Many people confuse an orgasm with ejaculation but the two are different. Generally, ejaculation is caused by the contraction of pelvic floor muscles, which has been induced by nerve stimulation. Ejaculations can happen when you are awake or asleep. A nocturnal emission or 'wet dream' is a combination of erotic stimulation during sleep combined with some limited amount of friction. This generally occurs in younger patients, and often in older men for a variety of reasons, including not having active intercourse or ejaculating on a regular basis.

Ejaculations that happen when you are awake need more physical stimulation than when you are asleep. The nervous system still stimulates the muscles, but it is more of a reflex response. When the bulbocavernosus muscles contract, an ejaculation occurs – this is when fluid is propelled out of your penis. Sometimes this gets referred to as an orgasm, but an orgasm is the actual contraction of these muscles expelling the fluid.

During ejaculation, the bladder neck closes and semen is expelled from the penis through the urethra. Semen consists of sperm produced in the testicles and fluid from the seminal vesicle and prostate gland.

It is possible to have an orgasm without the expelling of fluid ('anejaculation'). It is also possible to have the fluid go backwards into the bladder, which is called a 'retrograde ejaculation'. This is most commonly seen in men who have had prostate surgery, or surgery to the bladder neck or who have suffered a spinal cord injury (see section below).

Additionally, some men will have a failure of ejaculation. In other words, the fluid will not be deposited, and therefore, nothing will be ejaculated.

As you can see, there are numerous ejaculatory disorders, but the most common ejaculatory problem is rapid ejaculation (RE).

Rapid ejaculation

There are various textbook definitions of rapid ejaculation (RE). They range from ejaculation before vaginal, anal or oral entry, to any ejaculation occurring before both partners want it to happen. The general consensus is that rapid ejaculation is ejaculation occurring either before entry or within 30 seconds of entry of the vagina, anus or mouth.

My husband ejaculates within 2 minutes and then it is all over. He refuses to see a doctor because he feels it is normal. I don't have a problem getting an orgasm, but shouldn't a session last longer?

Sex doesn't have to last for any specific length of time, nor occur with any specific frequency, but needs to last for long enough and be often enough for the people involved in that sexual relationship to feel satisfied. If you and your husband are both satisfied with penetrative sex that lasts only a couple of moments, there is no need to seek help, as long as you are both happy about the situation. If you are unhappy, it may be that prolonging the foreplay or contact with him after he ejaculates will remedy the situation. If you decide to seek help, you could try counselling or drug treatments and you should discuss this with your local doctor or local sexual health specialist.

My erections are good, now that I am being prescribed Viagra, but I have noticed that I am ejaculating too quickly. This is causing me more distress than the impotence, as I have never suffered from this before. My partner now doesn't want to have sex, as she finds it frustrating because I ejaculate within seconds of me entering her. What can I do?

Your rapid ejaculation may be due to anxiety and fear of losing your erection. When men start to suffer from ED, they find that the erections gradually become weaker or they lose their erections quicker. Therefore men start to reduce the amount of foreplay they have and have penetrative sex quicker, and hence ejaculate quicker, before they lose the erection altogether to try and overcome the problem of ED. This happens frequently for men when they haven't been able to get an erection and now can. Most men in this situation, after they resume having regular sex, will learn how to control their ejaculation. If this doesn't happen for you and you continue to ejaculate before you wish to, then you need to speak to your doctor about this, either to get some information about different exercises you and your partner can do, or to have a different type of drug therapy.

My friend says he can delay his ejaculation for ages, and that his partner really likes this. Why can't I?

This is one of the most common questions asked by men, and particularly young men. The first thing to stress again is that sexual intercourse does not have to last any given length of time. It has to last long enough for a man and his sexual partner to be satisfied. Many men talk to their friends who say that they are able to delay ejaculation indefinitely and this leads to greater satisfaction in their partners. This is not always true and thinking that your own sexual performance has to be the same as other people's can be very unhelpful and in fact dangerous.

RE can also lead to a vicious cycle where the more you are concerned about it, the faster the ejaculation comes, which reinforces the original problem, and indeed can result in ejaculation without an erection. It is also true that there is a strong association between RE and ED. In some older men, the ejaculation can be triggered by a loss of erection during or immediately before intercourse.

What causes RE then?

Usually rapid ejaculation is due to psychological problems rather than physical. The psychological problems can include anxiety, guilt, difficulty in holding back ejaculate, and the 'haste' scenario. The haste scenario is a lifestyle problem, not having enough time or privacy. For example, when you were a teenager and you masturbated, you didn't know when somebody was going to enter your room; or, when you first started having sex, it was in the back of the car or whilst your partner's parents were out, and you never knew when they were coming back.

There are other sexual problems associated with RE. ED is frequently seen with RE especially in older men where the ejaculation is triggered by the failing erection. Loss of sex drive may be associated as a man may lose interest in sexual activity if he is embarrassed at the rapidity of his ejaculation. Another scenario is that the rapid ejaculation may be due to his partner's loss of interest in sex and an associated feeling of 'I may as well get this over quickly'.

If you are experiencing sexual difficulties or drinking too much alcohol, then this may be causing your RE. Alcohol-induced RE tends to happen occasionally rather than all the time.

Am I abnormal? I can't seem to last as long as the men do in the films?

It is hard to define what is normal. As long as you and your partner are satisfied with your lovemaking then that is all that matters.

Unfortunately a lot of men have learned all about ejaculation and sex from pornographic movies, where it is common to see men with sustained erections for long periods of time and ejaculations that appear to constitute a gallon of fluid. Pornographic movies might be useful in gaining knowledge and helping you become aroused but remember to take it at face value – you never know how many 'takes' were made to get that one clip!

Treatment

There are several treatment options: self-help, counselling or medication.

Are there any drugs that could help rapid ejaculation?

Drug therapy is based either on changing the sensation coming from the penis or on altering the way the mind perceives these sensations.

Drugs that would decrease the sensation coming from the penis include local anaesthetic creams such as lignocaine gel. The disadvantage is that sex is all about sensation and it is difficult to use these creams without numbing the penis and thus losing all sensation. The other major problem with them is that they can also numb the vagina, anus or mouth, thus taking away any sort of sensation for your partner.

The mainstay of drug therapy is to use antidepressants such as sertraline and clomipramine. These drugs can be taken either every night or prior to planned sexual activity. They are, however, drugs that can be obtained only on prescription, and you need to discuss with your doctor the advantages and disadvantages of a medication that affects not only the penis, but the entire body.

I don't really want to take drugs. Is there anything else that can help me?

Regarding treatment, like other sexual dysfunctions, the treatment options can be either counselling or therapy with drugs, or these two options can be combined. If you decide to go ahead with counselling, you will be offered a variety of techniques to try:

- **Behavioural techniques** for the management of rapid ejaculation rely on you recognizing when you are coming close to ejaculating, but before it becomes inevitable. One technique is the so-called '**stop-start method**'. This is where you know when you are nearing the point of losing voluntary control over ejaculation – you then stop any sort of stimulation, waiting until the urge has decreased. This method requires help and understanding from your partner, but can be very successful when used by a motivated couple.
- The second technique is the so-called '**squeeze technique**', which involves a man or his partner squeezing the end of the penis, again just before the point of inevitability. The penis needs to be squeezed quite hard between the thumb and the forefinger for about 4–5 seconds or until the sensation of ejaculation passes. Do this several times before allowing ejaculation to occur. It sounds easy to do but it takes a lot of practice. Some doctors recommend using distraction techniques, like counting backwards etc.

but you are there to enjoy yourself not to think about what jobs need doing around the house, so stay focused on what you are doing and you will be able to recognize the stage in the orgasm prior to ejaculation.

- There is another technique called 'sensate focus', which is described in Chapter 6.

I am gay and suffer from rapid ejaculation and my boyfriend and I are getting very frustrated as it is ruining our sexual relationship, which is very important to both of us. I don't want to bother my GP with it, so is there anything that I can do myself?

You can learn to recognize the stage in the orgasm cycle prior to ejaculation, but before it is inevitable, and prevent ejaculation by using the squeeze technique (see question above).

My doctor suggested that I use anaesthetic creams to help my RE. Are there any herbal anaesthetic creams?

There is limited research into herbal products that help to control rapid ejaculation. There are some over-the-counter anaesthetic creams (but not herbal) that have been successfully used to treat rapid ejaculation. You would need to apply roughly half a teaspoon of anaesthetic cream to the penis approximately 30 minutes before sexual relations are initiated. Treatment could be successful, but an obvious side effect is vaginal, anal or oral anaesthesia (i.e. a lack of sensation for your partner). Make sure your partner is not allergic to the creams beforehand.

No ejaculation

It is important to distinguish between two issues here. Some men do not have the sensation of reaching orgasm, while others complain of reaching orgasm but there being no ejaculate emitted.

The two most common causes of not reaching orgasm are psychological or prescription medication. If you were able to ejaculate in the past, without pain, but now find you can't and you haven't had any of the physical problems or prescription medication mentioned below, then your problem could be due to psychological reasons. Talk to your doctor who will help you identify and address the causes and refer you to a specialist if necessary.

Many prescription drugs can delay or prevent orgasm, such or antidepressants (e.g. paroxetine and amitriptyline). The ability to reach orgasm may return to normal when you stop taking the medication, but **never** stop taking medication until you have discussed it with your doctor first.

If you get an orgasm but no ejaculate, you may be suffering from what is called 'retrograde' ejaculation; this can occur when the bladder neck fails to close and semen passes into the bladder rather than coming out of the penis. It can be due to physical reasons or prescribed medication, such as those that treat high blood pressure (e.g. methyldopa), alpha blockers (which may be taken to treat symptoms of prostate enlargement), or cold medications. Up to 90% of men have no ejaculation following surgery for prostate problems. The most common surgery is transurethral resection of the prostate (TURP). The cause is damage to the bladder neck. Other conditions may also cause retrograde ejaculation, such as spina bifida, diabetes and neurological diseases.

As you get older, it is perfectly normal not to pass so much ejaculate.

My GP has told me I suffer from retrograde ejaculation and there is no need to refer me to a specialist. Why?

If you and your partner are trying for a baby, you will need to seek medical advice, but there is no other reason to be referred to a specialist unless you have other symptoms.

Retrograde ejaculation will not affect your health. Your semen will leave your bladder when you next pass urine.

If I have retrograde ejaculation what can done about it ?

There are various ways of helping the problem:

- You could reduce your dose of alpha blockers if you have been prescribed these. Discuss this first with your doctor.
- Drugs such as imipramine might help.
- You can try having intercourse with a full bladder.

My fiancé, who is in the army and just back from two tours abroad, seems to have developed a problem with climaxing. He has no problem getting an erection and can stimulate himself to orgasm, but he can't climax through intercourse. He wonders if masturbating frequently when he was away has caused this problem. What can we do?

Masturbation has been discouraged over the centuries by a variety of tales attributing various physical side effects to it, such as blindness. However, with the liberalization of sexual attitudes, doctors now realize that masturbation is a very common form of sexual activity and carries with it no stigma or physical side effects. However, the social stigma can lead to psychological side effects, which can in turn lead to sexual dysfunction. The phenomenon that your fiancé is suffering from is known as secondary 'anorgasmia'. (Primary anorgasmia is a very rare condition and occurs in men who have never been able to ejaculate. This is caused by failure of the male ejaculatory mechanisms to develop properly.) Secondary anorgasmia is far more likely to be of psychological origin and can develop for a variety of reasons. There are many possible treatment routes open to you and your fiancé, including psychosexual counselling (see Chapter 6). If infertility is the major problem and it cannot be overcome by counselling, you will need to see a specialist to discuss methods of assisted conception.

My sexual problem is that I cannot reach orgasm. What causes this?

If you have trouble reaching orgasm at all, the two most common reasons for this are either a side effect of drug therapy, or psychological issues interrupting the ejaculatory process. Regarding drug therapy, many commonly used drugs cause delay or absence of orgasm. These include social drugs such as alcohol, marijuana, cocaine and methadone, as well as prescription drugs such as the anxiolytic medications (Prozac and amitriptyline), blood pressure drugs (methyldopa and thiazide diuretics). If you think that it is one of the medications that you are on causing your sexual problem, please discuss this with your doctor; **don't** stop your medication without discussing this issue with your doctor first.

Psychological issues are a very common cause of all sexual dysfunctions in men. A lack of orgasm can be associated with, for instance, a very strict upbringing, religious beliefs about loss of semen or from repeated efforts at 'stop-start' sex.

My problem is that I feel that I have an orgasm, but nothing comes out.

If this has always been the case, it may be that you have a very rare failure of the ejaculatory system to develop. You will need to discuss this with your doctor and be referred to see a specialist urologist. However, far more frequently, this problem develops in a man in later life, and can be due to a variety of causes. The most common is traumatic, particularly after bladder neck incision or prostatectomy or other pelvic surgery. This then causes retrograde ejaculation where the semen, rather than coming out when a man ejaculates, occurs backwards into the bladder. A similar problem can occur more rarely after an infection or from a stone in the ejaculatory duct, or after spinal cord injury.

It is very common as men get older for the volume of ejaculate to decrease. This is not suggestive of any specific disease.

If you are using any of the drugs mentioned earlier, reduction of these may help the situation. If they have been prescribed by your doctor, **don't reduce them yourself**, but discuss the problem with your doctor. If there is no obvious cause, then you may benefit from seeing a psychosexual counsellor.

When I have sex with my partner, I have the feeling that I have an orgasm but don't ejaculate. Is this normal? I had a spinal cord injury 2 years ago.

Yes. If your spinal cord injury (SCI) is in the lower part of your back, then it can inhibit you from ejaculating, and this is called retrograde ejaculation. Ejaculation is a motor function which cannot take place if you have damaged nerves and parts of the spinal cord that control ejaculation. Men with SCI who do ejaculate may experience retrograde ejaculation. Orgasm does not necessarily accompany ejaculation. Because of sensory loss, few SCI men are able to reach and experience the type of orgasm that they had before their injury. Heightened spasticity has also been experienced by some men at the point of ejaculation.

Not all SCI men attempt having sex, for whatever reason. However, for those who do, many are successful.

Regarding drug therapy, many commonly used drugs cause delay or absence of orgasm. These include social drugs such as alcohol, marijuana, cocaine and methadone, as well as prescription drugs such as the anxiolytic medications (Prozac and amitriptyline), blood pressure drugs (methyldopa and thiazide diuretics). If you think that it is one of the medications that you are on causing your sexual problem, please discuss this with your doctor; **don't** stop your medication without discussing this issue with your doctor.

Blood in sperm

I've got blood in my ejaculate. Should I go and see my GP?

Blood in your ejaculate is usually nothing to worry about – it is a condition called 'haematospermia'. It is usually due to inflammation of the seminal vesicles (the structure that stores fluid prior to ejaculation), or the prostate. Antibiotics will easily treat this condition, and it is rarely associated with a something nasty, like cancer. A careful examination by a doctor can rule out this possibility.

12
Peyronie's disease

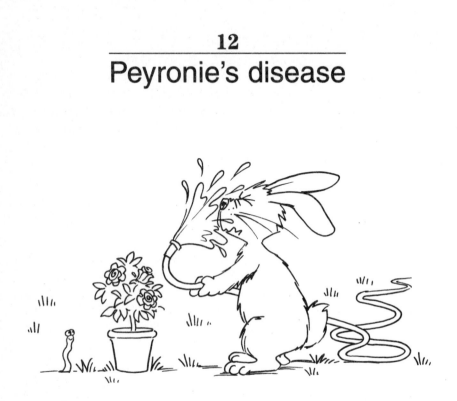

A French physician named François Gigot de la Peyronie first described Peyronie's disease in 1743. He reported that scar tissue (a fibrotic and sometimes calcified plaque under the skin of the penis) caused a significant bend in his patients' penises (Figure 12.1), most evident when the penis was erect. Until recently, Peyronie's disease was a poorly understood condition. It can affect all men regardless of age, as young as 18 years, but it is more common in men aged between 40 and 60 occurring in 0.5–1% of this age group.

This scarring often results in pain on erection, curvature of the penis during erection and a lump that can be felt in the shaft of the penis. Your ability to have proper intercourse depends on the degree of curvature in the penis – if the curvature increases to a severe angle, sexual intercourse may become uncomfortable for both partners or even impossible. The scarring can range from a few millimetres or may encompass the entire length of the penis. Patients often delay seeking medical help out of fear and embarrassment and it can sometimes subside without treatment anyway. The most common reason for seeking medical help is painful erections and ED.

The disease is associated with other similar conditions including Dupuytren's contracture where the tendons in the hand shrink, and there are small fibrotic plaques in the palm of the hand, causing the fingers to be permanently bent – this is present in 10–25% of Peyronie's disease cases.

What causes Peyronie's disease?

The causes are poorly understood. Currently, a number of theories seem to indicate that trauma is the most likely cause. It

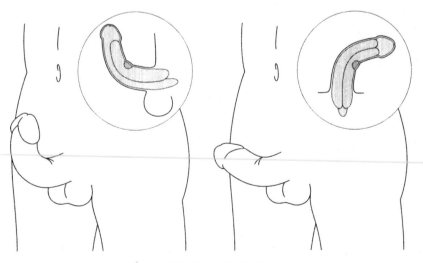

Figure 12.1 Peyronie's disease.

was once thought that masturbation or sexually transmitted diseases would produce scarring, but this is just a myth. Peyronie's disease results from injury followed by scarring.

Unfortunately, as with most things relating to human sexuality, we are not taught how to have sex. Consequently, many positions that young men practise can put a great deal of twisting pressure on the penis, causing trauma to its delicate supportive structures. Whenever there is damage, scar tissue develops and restricts the blood flow to the area. It either impedes the blood flow, causing ED, or it causes a bending in the penis at the level of the scar.

Other suggestions for possible causes include a possible genetic connection, changes in the blood vessels associated with hardening of the arteries, infection and diabetes.

Peyronie's disease has also been associated with certain medications such as beta blockers, the drugs often used in the treatment of high blood pressure.

I have read about Peyronie's disease quite by chance in the newspapers and I am worried that I may have it. What signs would I have if I did have Peyronie's disease?

The diagnosis of Peyronie's disease is based on whether you have all three signs of pain, plaque formation and bending of the penis on erection. The pain occurs in approximately 60–70% of men with the disease, but this almost always gets better by itself after a few months, with only 10% of men having pain lasting longer than 2 years. Most men first notice the typical hardened area within the penis (called 'plaque'). The commonest site is on the shaft of the penis on the upper surface, but it can occur anywhere on the penis and indeed there may be more than one place affected.

It is important to remember that the disease takes 12–18 months to fully develop, at which stage the bend in the penis may change. It is often associated with ED. Go and see your doctor as soon as you feel any pain or abnormal lumps in your penis. If Peyronie's disease is diagnosed, ask your doctor to explain about the condition and the treatment options that are available. If your doctor is unable to answer your questions, request a referral to a consultant with a special interest in male sexual health problems.

In about 13% of men, the disease will clear by itself, but this may take several years. However, there are treatments available and the sooner the condition is treated the earlier it can be helped.

With that description, I think I do have Peyronie's disease. What should I do?

If you have pain in your penis, or you can feel a lump, or the penis is bent to an extent that makes intercourse difficult, then you should speak about this to your GP. Note, however, that most penises are bent slightly either to the left, or the right, or up or down, and it is only if this is an increasing problem, or there is pain associated with it, that you need to see your doctor about it.

If your GP confirms the diagnosis, he will refer you to the local urologist, who is a specialist in disorders of the urinary tract. Tests may include an injection into your penis to establish an erection so that the bend of your penis can be measured and perhaps recorded by photography.

I have a lot of pain in my penis. What can I do to help this?

You can take simple painkillers, such as soluble aspirin or paracetamol, for this pain, as long as you have no other medical problems that would stop you taking these medications. However, if pain persists, then it is important that you go along to your GP or to a genitourinary medicine clinic – this branch of medicine studies and treats problems in your reproductive and urinary organs. The doctors here should be able to diagnose accurately the cause of the pain in your penis.

My penis is bent and it is uncomfortable for my partner when we have sex. Should we try different positions?

This question raises several issues. Your partner might indeed have pain because of the bend in your penis. This can be overcome by trying different positions in order to attempt to find one where you both feel comfortable and does not cause either you or your partner pain; for instance you could try lying underneath instead of on top, or lying side by side.

However, the pain that she is having associated with sex may not be due to the bend in your penis at all. She needs to talk to her GP or gynaecologist in order to make sure that there are no other problems going on that are making intercourse painful for her. If she has already undergone the menopause, then one of the commonest causes of pain with intercourse is the vagina becoming relatively drier than it was when she was younger, and you and your partner could use some vaginal lubrication to assist during intercourse, such as K-Y Jelly or Sensilube.

Treatment

I have now been told that I have Peyronie's disease. Have I just got to put up with it or is there anything that can be done for me?

It is important to remember that many men with Peyronie's disease do not require any treatment. Over the years a large number of treatments have been used, but no single treatment has been shown to be effective in all cases.

In the early stages, tamoxifen (taken by mouth) has been shown to produce an improvement by preventing the formation of fibrous plaque. (Although this drug is also given for the treatment of breast cancer, the two conditions are not related.)

Vitamin E is a simple and sometimes effective way to ease the pain and deformity of the disease. It will not alter any underlying erectile dysfunction.

Verapamil, a calcium channel blocker often used in the treatment of hypertension, has been shown to decrease the plaque size and pain in Peyronie's disease when injected directly into the plaque. Other treatments include colchicine, potaba and interferon.

There have been recent trials in the treatment of Peyronie's with extracorporeal shock wave therapy (ESWT) and, although initial results have been promising, as yet the long-term outcome is to be determined.

Unfortunately, at this time there is no real cure for Peyronie's disease. Like many problems in medicine, when it is not known exactly what the cause is, there could be several potential treatments, some of which work for some people. Chatting to your GP will help to find the best solution for you – he or she will talk about the pros and cons of the different treatments available.

I have tried all sorts of things for Peyronie's disease. Could I have surgery to correct the problem?

If your problem has remained unchanged for over 6 months, surgery is an option but there is no 'best' operation. Before a doctor will refer you for surgery, the disease should have remained unchanged for over 6 months. This avoids surgery on someone whose problem might sort itself. About 10% of patients will find surgery necessary if the deformity is such that it prevents sexual intercourse.

Surgery is normally offered only to those who have difficulty inserting the penis during intercourse. If you are still able to enjoy sexual intercourse, even though you have a bend in your penis, then surgery won't be recommended.

The basis of the surgery is to take out the plaque in the penis. This area can then either be replaced by a graft of a patient's own vein or a synthetic substance. Alternatively, a small area can be taken out from the other side of your penis to straighten it out. This operation, called the 'Nesbit procedure', is regarded as the gold standard for surgical treatment of Peyronie's disease. A penis with a substantial bend has segments taken out from the opposite side to the fibrous plaque, to create a straight penis. As with all operations, this has complications:

- Difficulty with erections can occur after the operation.
- The bend to the opposite side might be overcorrected.
- Scarring can develop.
- The glans or the shaft of the penis can become numb.

- The penis can shorten.
- The wound can become infected.

The operation doesn't remove the plaque; tissues are merely removed from the opposite side. However, the procedure is successful in 80% of men and you will be able to have sexual intercourse 4 weeks after surgery.

There are other operative procedures, with their own advantages and disadvantages. Ask your doctor for a referral to a consultant about the variety of available operations.

This all sounds rather drastic! Would a prosthesis help?

A prosthesis for your penis would i nvolve another operation to repair this condition, but it would indeed not only straighten your penis but improve erections as well. Talk to your GP about these possibilities.

What can I do to help myself?

Find out as much as you can about the disease and the treatments. If you feel that your GP is unable to help, there are clinics as previously mentioned, where you can get advice. Support and understanding from your partner is a great help and relieve a lot of the worries and pressure.

Remember, the disease is not linked to infections or cancer. The main aim is to treat the condition and correct the deformity, which may take a while.

Glossary

alprostadil A drug based on the hormone-like substance prostaglandin. It is most commonly used as an injection into the penis to help produce an erection.

anus The 'back passage'.

anejaculation The inability to ejaculate.

angioplasty Surgery to reconstruct the blood vessels damaged by disease or injury.

anorgasmia The failure to reach orgasm.

aphrodisiac Any substance that stimulates sexual desire.

artery Any blood vessel that carries blood from the heart to another part of the body.

artery hardening Uneven thickening of the inside of some artery walls. Caused by fatty deposits from the blood, which harden with time. Largely the result of a persistently unhealthy diet, and eventually leading to blood circulation problems.

benign tumour A non-invading, or non-malignant, tumour.

bladder The urinary bladder is the sac situated in the front of the pelvis that stores urine before its expulsion from the body via the urethra. The bladder wall is composed largely of smooth muscle tissue and expands as urine flows into it from the kidneys via the ureters.

bladder neck The part of the bladder next to the upper surface of the prostate gland.

bulbocavernosus muscles Muscles in the pelvis.

chronic Long-lasting (often permanent) disease or condition.

corpora cavernosa The two largest of the three major columns of tissue within the penis. They sit on either side of the penis and together form the main part of the erect penis, filling with blood during sexual stimulation.

corpus spongiosum This is the third major and middle column of tissue within the penis and also the part of the penis that protects the urethra on its passage out of the body; it enlarges to form the 'glans' or tip of the penis.

diabetes This is an increasingly common disease, and it comes in varying degrees of severity. Essentially, diabetes is a metabolic disorder resulting in too much sugar in the blood and characterized by the excretion of large quantities of urine.

dialysis (haemodialysis) This is a common treatment for kidney failure involving filtering blood through a membrane that acts as a kind of artificial kidney, removing impurities and waste products.

dyspareunia Painful intercourse.

ejaculation The expulsion of semen out of the penis through the urethra. Ejaculation is caused by contraction of the pelvic muscles lying just behind the penis.

endocrine Anything related to the body's hormones.

erectile dysfunction (ED) A persistent inability to produce or maintain an erection sufficient to achieve the kind of sex desired by a man and his partner.

erection The hardening of the penis. An erection happens when the erectile tissue of the penis becomes engorged with blood.

Fibrosis The formation of an excessive amount of fibrous tissue in a body organ or part – usually as a result of inflammation, irritation or healing.

fibrous Consisting of, containing or resembling fibres. Often used to describe tissue that has hardened and contracted.

flaccid Lacking firmness or rigidity – soft and limp. Often used to describe the penis in its non-aroused state.

genital Anything related to the reproductive or sexual organs (e.g. the penis) of the male or female.

genitourinary Anything related to either the reproductive or the excretory (urinary) organs of the male or female. Genitourinary medicine is the branch of medical science concerned with the study and treatment of diseases of these organs, including sexually transmitted diseases.

glans The bulbous tip or 'head' of the penis.

haematospermia Blood in the sperm.

hormone A chemical produced by the body that affects its everyday function. Testosterone, for example, is a hormone that controls sexual desire.

impotence See erectile dysfunction.

impregnate To make pregnant.

infertility An inability to have children (i.e. sterile rather than fertile). Infertility may be due to factors in the male or the female partner, or both. Not to be confused with impotence.

libido Sexual urge or desire.

malignant Likely to cause harm or damage. Often used to refer to a tumour or cancer that is resistant to treatment and possibly life-threatening. Opposite to benign.

morning erection The erection that normally occurs as part of the waking-up process in healthy men. It is caused subconsciously by the warmth of being in bed and often also associated with the need to pass urine. It is usually present on waking but disappears shortly afterwards or on passing urine.

multiple sclerosis A chronic progressive disease of the central nervous system. Associated with speech and sight problems, a lack of coordination, tremor and some paralysis. In young men, ED may be the only symptom of multiple sclerosis, so GPs should be aware of the association.

neurological Anything related to the nervous system (which controls the muscles and also monitors sensations around the body).

organic When used to describe a cause of ED, it means that the cause is physical, i.e. associated with other body functions or, more accurately, dysfunctions.

parasympathetic nervous system The part of the nervous system responsible for relaxation.

pelvic Relating to the pelvis – the basin-shaped part of the skeleton situated between the torso and the legs (and including the hips in humans).

penile prosthesis In general terms, a prosthesis is an artificial substitute for a missing part. A prosthesis for the penis is more an implant than a replacement, however, most commonly consisting of two firm rods inserted inside the penis shaft.

persistent Long-lasting or continuous.

Peyronie's disease Associated with two symptoms of pain inside the shaft and a bend along the shaft of the penis. Both symptoms are the result of inflammation inside the shaft of the penis, which may have occurred for a number of reasons. Surgery can help to correct the bend in Peyronie's disease.

placebo Harmless or inactive substance administered in the same way as a drug or medicine, usually in research, to help distinguish the true effectiveness of a drug or medicine.

placebo effect A positive therapeutic effect claimed by a patient after receiving a placebo, in the false belief that the placebo that they received was actually an active drug.

priapism Prolonged erection (4 hours or more). Can often occur because a treatment for ED has worked too well. Requires urgent medical treatment.

prostate gland A small, conical gland that surrounds the neck of the bladder at its base just in front of the rectum (in men only), and secretes the liquid part of the semen (which becomes the seminal fluid).

prostaglandin A potent, hormone-like substance found in many body tissues, and in the semen, and often used in injections to treat ED.

psychogenic Originating in the mind, rather than the body (i.e. of psychological, rather than physical, origin).

psychosexual Anything related to the mental or psychological aspects of sex – sexual fantasies, for example.

rapid ejaculation Ejaculation too soon – the accepted definition is 'ejaculation before or within 30 seconds of insertion of the penis into the partner', but a more appropriate definition is 'whenever a man feels that he ejaculates too soon or has lost control of his ejaculation'.

renal Relating to the kidneys and urine excretion.

retrograde ejaculation Occurs when semen is forced backwards into the bladder during orgasm, instead of being forced outwards and expelled from the body.

self-esteem Self-respect, or a high or positive opinion of oneself. Lack of self-esteem is common in men who are unable to have normal erections and is often expressed as a feeling of worthlessness.

semen The thick, whitish fluid produced during ejaculation. It contains the sperm.

seminal fluid Fluid produced largely by the prostate gland, but finally by the seminal vesicles, which, together with sperm, makes up semen. Seminal fluid is essential for a successful pregnancy.

seminal vesicle Small pouch between the testicles and penis, which finally prepares and stores the semen before ejaculation.

sensate focus A type of psychological therapy that encourages a couple to relax in each other's company (again) before they attempt to resume a sexual relationship.

shaft Any elongated cylindrical structure. In this context, the main part of the erect penis.

side effect Any effect of a drug or treatment other than the main or desired effect (but usually used to describe an unwanted additional effect).

specialist A person who devotes him or herself to a particular activity or field – in this context, usually a hospital-based doctor who has specialized (compared to a GP, who is a general doctor) in genitourinary medicine, urology, or psychiatry.

sperm The part of the semen that enables a man to make his female partner pregnant.

surgery Incision to investigate or remove a body part, rather than treatment with drugs or other medication.

sympathetic nervous system The part of the nervous system responsible for excitation.

testosterone A strong hormone that controls sexual desire. It is secreted mainly by the testicles and is responsible for the secondary sexual characteristics of men (e.g. facial hair).

therapy Another word for treatment.

tunica albuginea The tough, outer layer of each of the corpora cavernosa. Once the corpora cavernosa have filled up with blood (during an erection), the tunica albuginea stops it all draining away.

urethra The tube that passes through the penis from the bladder, which is normally used to excrete urine, but is also used to ejaculate semen during orgasm.

urological Anything related to a disorder or illness of the urinary tract (urethra).

urologist A doctor who specializes in disorders and surgical treatment of the urinary tract.

vagina Part of the female reproductive tract, where the penis is inserted for sexual intercourse.

vaginal containment The third and final stage of sensate focus therapy, during which the man is allowed to penetrate his partner, but neither partner is allowed to move. Once this stage can be maintained without the man losing his erection, the couple can progress to movement and orgasm and ejaculation.

vaginismus Involuntary contractions of the muscles surrounding the vagina.

Appendix 1
Useful addresses

Age Concern England
Astral House
1268 London Road
London SW16 4ER
Tel: 020 8765 7200

**British Association of
Counselling and
Psychotherapy**
1 Regent Place
Rugby CV21 2PJ
Tel: 0870 443 5252
Website: www.bcc.co.uk

**British Association for
Sexual and Relationship
Therapy**
PO Box 13686,
London SW20 9ZH

Couple Counselling Scotland
40 North Castle Street
Edinburgh EH2 3BN
Tel: 0131 225 5006
Website: www.couplecounselling.org

Diabetes UK
(Formerly British Diabetic
Association)
10 Parkway
London NW1 7AA
Tel: 020 7424 1000
Fax: 020 7424 1001
Careline: 020 7424 1030 (voice)
020 7424 1888 (text)
Website: www.diabetes.org.uk

Family Planning Association
2–12 Pentonville Road
London N1 9FP
Tel: 020 7837 5432
Website: www.fpa.org.uk

Health Development Agency
(Formerly Health Education
Authority)
Trevelyan House
30 Great Peter Street
London SW1P 2HW
Tel: 020 7222 5300
Website: www.hda-online.org.uk

Impotence Association
see Sexual Dysfunction
Association

Institute of Psychosexual Medicine
12 Chandos Street
Cavendish Square
London W1M 9DE
Tel: 020 7580 0631
Website: www.ipm.org.uk

Jewish Marriage Council
23 Ravenhurst Avenue
London NW4 4EE
Tel: 020 8203 6311

Marriage Care
(previously Catholic Marriage
Advisory Centre)
Clitherow House
1 Blythe Mews
Blythe Road
London W14 0NW
Helpline: 0845 757 3921

Multiple Sclerosis Society of Great Britain and Northern Ireland
The MS National Centre
372 Edgeware Road
London NW2 6ND
Helpline: 0808 800 8000
Tel: 020 8438 0700
Website: www.mssociety.org.uk

Owen Mumford Ltd
Brook Hill
Woodstock
Oxford OX20 1TU
Helpline: 0800 731 6959
Tel: 01993 813 466
Website: www.owenmumford.com

Parkinson's Disease Society
National Office
215 Vauxhall Bridge Road
London SW1V 1EJ
Tel: 020 7931 8080
Fax: 020 7233 9908
Helpline: 0808 800 0303
Website: www.parkinsons.org.uk

RELATE
(England headquarters)
Herbert Gray College
Little Church Street
Rugby CV21 3AP
Tel: 01788 573 241
Website: www.relate.org.uk

Spinal Injuries Association
76 St James Lane
London N10 3DF
Helpline: 0800 980 0501
Tel: 020 8444 2121
Website: www.spinal.co.uk

Sexual Dysfunction Association
PO Box 10296
London SW17 9WH
Helpline: 020 8767 7791
Website: www.impotence.org.uk

SPOD (Association to Aid the Sexual and Personal Relationships of People with a Disability)
286 Camden Road
London N7 0BJ
Tel: 020 7607 8851
Website: www.spod-uk.org

Appendix 2
Useful publications

Books by Class Publishing

Diabetes – the 'at your fingertips' guide (5th edition)
   by Professor Peter Sönksen, Dr Charles Fox and Sue Judd
   Published by Class Publishing, London 2001, ISBN 1 85959 087 X
Heart Health – the 'at your fingertips' guide (2nd edition)
   by Dr Graham Jackson
   Published by Class Publishing, London 2000, ISBN 1 85959 009 8
High Blood Pressure – the 'at your fingertips' guide (2nd edition)
   by Dr Julian Tudor Hart and Dr Tom Fahey
   Published by Class Publishing, London 1999, ISBN 1 872362 81 8
Kidney: Dialysis and Transplants – the 'at your fingertips' guide
   by Dr Andy Stein and Janet Wild
   Published by Class Publishing, London 2002, ISBN 1 85959 046 2
Multiple Sclerosis – the 'at your fingertips' guide
   by Professor Ian Robinson, Dr Stuart Neilson and Dr Frank
   Clifford Rose
   Published by Class Publishing, London 2000, ISBN 1 872362 94 X
Parkinson's – the 'at your fingertips' guide (2nd edition)
   by Dr Marie Oxtoby and Dr Adrian Williams
   Published by Class Publishing, London 2002, ISBN 1 872362 96 6

Other books on erectile dysfunction

The Haynes Man Manual. The practical step-by-step guide to men's health
by Ian Banks
Published by Haynes Manuals. ISBN 1 85960 931 7
Impotence: a guide for men of all ages
by Wallace Dinsmore and Philip Kell
Published by the Royal Society of Medicine Press Ltd,
London 2002, ISBN 1 85315 402 4
Erectile dysfunction – clinical drawings for your patients
by Christine M Evans and Philip Kell
Published by Health Press, Oxford 2000, ISBN 1 899541 11 X
Erectile dysfunction: fast facts (2nd edition)
by Roger Kirby, Simon Holmes and Professor Culley Carson
Published by Health Press, Oxford 1998, ISBN 1 899541 47 0
Impotence
by Michael Foster and Martin Cole
Published by Martin Dunitz Publishers, London 1996,
ISBN 1 85317 329 0
The Which? *guide to men's health* (3rd edition)
by Dr Steve Carroll
Published by Which? Ltd, London 1999, ISBN 0 85202 758 3

Website

A comprehensive list of treatments for impotence is maintained by
the Impotence World Association at www.impotenceworld.org. Drugs are
often called by different names in the USA, so you may need the
help of your doctor to interpret them.

Index

Have you found **Sexual Health for Men – the at your fingertips'
guide** useful and practical? If so, you may be interested in other
books from Class Publishing.

High Blood Pressure – the 'at your fingertips' guide
SECOND EDITION £14.99
*Dr Julian Tudor Hart, Dr Tom Fahey
and Professor Wendy Savage*
The authors use all their years of
experience as blood pressure
experts to answer over 340 real
questions on high blood pressure.

Heart Health – the 'at your fingertips' guide
SECOND EDITION £14.99
Dr Graham Jackson
This practical handbook, written by a
leading cardiologist, answers all your
questions about heart conditions,
and tells you all about you and your
heart and how to make it as strong
as possible.

Kidney Dialysis and Transplants – the 'at your fingertips' guide
NEW TITLE £14.99
*Dr Andy Stein and Janet Wild
with Juliet Auer*
A practical handbook for anyone with
long-term kidney failure or their
families, offering positive, clear and
medically accurate advice on every
aspect of living with the condition.

Beating Depression – the 'at your fingertips' guide
£14.99
*Dr Stefan Cembrowicz
and Dr Dorcas Kingham*
Depression is one of most common
illnesses in the world – affecting up
to one in four people at some time in
their lives. *Beating Depression*
shows sufferers and their families
that they are not alone, and offers
tried and tested techniques for
overcoming depression.

Stroke – the 'at your fingertips' guide
£14.99
*Dr Anthony Rudd, Penny Irwin
and Bridget Penhale*
This essential guidebook tells you all
about strokes – most importantly
how to recover from them. The book
is full of practical advice, including
recuperation plans; you will find it
inspiring.

Cancer – the 'at your fingertips' guide
THIRD EDITION £14.99
*Val Speechley and Maxine
Rosenfield*
This invaluable reference guide gives
you clear and practical information
about cancer. You will find in this
book the information you need to
reassure yourself, and enable you to
take control.

Kidney Failure Explained
NEW SECOND EDITION £14.99
Dr Andy Stein and Janet Wild
The complete and updated reference
manual for people suffering from
kidney failure, telling you everything
you need to know about the
condition.

Stop that heart attack!
SECOND EDITION £14.99
Dr Derrick Cutting
The easy, drug-free and medically
accurate way to cut your risk of
having a heart attack dramatically.

Multiple Sclerosis – the 'at your fingertips' guide
*Ian Robinson, Dr Stuart Neilson
and Dr Frank Clifford Rose* £14.99
Straightforward and positive answers
to all your questions on MS.

PRIORITY ORDER FORM

Cut out or photocopy this form and send it (post free in the UK) to:

Class Publishing Priority Service
FREEPOST
London W6 7BR

Please send me urgently
(tick boxes below)

Post included
price per copy (UK only)

☐ **Sexual Health for Men – the 'at your fingertips' guide** £17.99
(ISBN 1 85959 011 X)

☐ **High Blood Pressure – the 'at your fingertips' guide** £17.99
(ISBN 1 872362 81 8)

☐ **Heart Health – the 'at your fingertips' guide** £17.99
(ISBN 1 85959 009 8)

☐ **Kidney Dialysis and Transplants – the 'at your fingertips' guide** £17.99
(ISBN 1 85959 046 2)

☐ **Beating Depression – the 'at your fingertips' guide** £17.99
(ISBN 1 85959 063 2)

☐ **Stroke – the 'at your fingertips' guide** £17.99
(ISBN 1872362 98 2)

☐ **Cancer – the 'at your fingertips' guide** £17.99
(ISBN 1 85959 036 5)

☐ **Kidney Failure Explained** £17.99
(ISBN 1 85959 070 5)

☐ **Stop that heart attack!** £17.99
(ISBN 1 85959 055 1)

☐ **Multiple Sclerosis – the 'at your fingertips' guide** £17.99
(ISBN 1 872362 94 X)

TOTAL _____

Easy ways to pay

Cheque: I enclose a cheque payable to Class Publishing for £ _____

Credit card: Please debit my

☐ Mastercard   ☐ Visa   ☐ Amex   ☐ Switch

Number _____ Expiry date _____

Name _____

My address for delivery is _____

_____

Town _____ County _____ Postcode _____

Telephone number (*in case of query*) _____

Credit card billing address if different from above _____

_____

Town _____ County _____ Postcode _____

Class Publishing's guarantee: remember that if, for any reason, you are not satisfied with these books, we will refund all your money, without any questions asked. Prices and VAT rates may be altered for reasons beyond our control.